# A GUIDE TO BODY PAINS

Attention Readers:

Every effort is made to ensure accuracy of material, but the publisher, printer and author will not be held responsible for any inadvertent error (s). In case of any dispute, all legal matters to be settled under Delhi Jurisdiction only.
Please consult an expert before strating any medication

*Published by*
*Lotus Press*

# A GUIDE TO BODY PAINS

**Dr. Rajeev Sharma**
*M.D., D.Lit.*

Lotus PRESS
4263/3, Ansari Road,
Darya Ganj, New Delhi-110002

**Lotus Press**
4263/3, Ansari Road, Darya Ganj, New Delhi- 110002
Ph.: 32903912, 23280047, E-mail: lotus_press@sify.com
www.lotuspress.co.in

**A GUIDE TO BODY PAINS**

ISBN: 81-8382-065-4



*Published by:* Lotus Press, New Delhi-110 002.
*Laser Typeset by:* Computek System, Delhi
*Printed at:* Nisha Enterprises, Delhi.

## A Brief About Dr. Rajeev Sharma

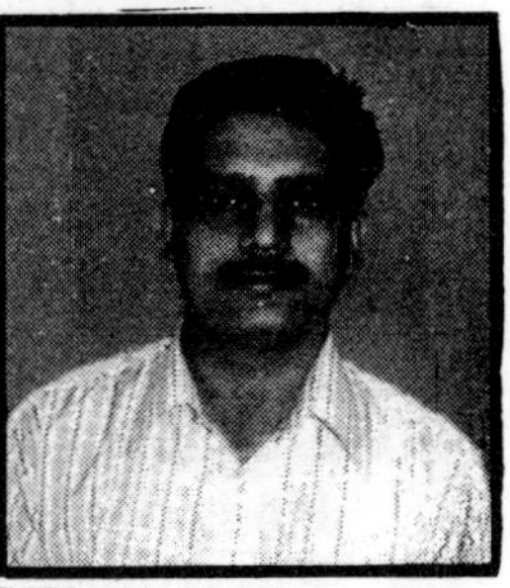

Dr. Rajeev Sharma is an eminent consultant of Homoeopathy, Yoga, Naturopathy and Alternative Medicine in India. He has written more than two hundred books (200) in Hindi and English and around one thousand articles which have been published in various newspapers and magazines. He is also an Editiorial Board Member of the prestigious *Asian Homoeopathic Journal* besides many other newspapers and magazines.

Dr. Rajeev Sharma has written books on ayurveda, allopathy, homoeopathy, yoga, naturopahty, accupressure, magnetotherapy, reiki, water-therapy, massage and aromatherapy etc.

The books written by Dr. Rajeev Sharma are published by renowned publishers of India. Besides this he is doing editing and translation also. He is content provider to many magazines.

Dr. Rajeev Sharma has written books on all major ailments like diabetes, hypertension, obesity, stomach and respiratiory disorders, E.N.T. disorders, female disorders, UTI disorders, paediatric problems, head ache, stress and other mental problems and Sexual Disorders etc. You can fix an appointment for any of such problem.

Dr. Rajeev Sharma is Medical Advisor to Ralson

Remedies (a homoeopathic drug manufacturer), and Dixit Pharmacy (Ayurvedic Manufacturer), Medical Examiner at the LIC and Medical Officer in U.P. Govt. He has received several prizes for his outstanding achievements. He has been awarded the *Best Author prize in Hindi* by the Ministry of Health and Family Welfare, Government of India and *Sarjana Puraskar by U.P. Hindi Sansthan,* Lucknow. He has delivered talks on All India Radio and lectures on Alternative Medicine in various Government and Non-government Organisations. He has written Advt. Scripts for the products of several companies.

He is working as Vastu Fengshui Consultant, Educational Consultant and Marriage and Behaviour Counsellor too.

He is delivering lectures and providing literature on Personality Development and Life Style Management also to the MNC's.

*He has established an institute through which you can get certificates by correspondence in Accupressure, Massage, Yoga, Water Therapy, Diet Therapy, Naturopathy, Colour Therapy and Reiki besides other paramedical courses.*

Dr. Rajeev Sharma is also a social activist. He has worked a lot against Addition and prevention of AIDS. Now a days, he is working to check the population growth of India with an NGO called 'Nav Chetna Manch'. He has worked for pollution control and human rights too and has received the World Human Rights Promotion Award. His name has been published in *LIMCA BOOK OF RECORDS* 2005. He has developed two websites too :-

www.newkamasutra.com : A site of love, romance and sex.
www.indiaalive.net : Patriotic site (Future planning)
He is a person of creative mind.

# PREFACE

Pains are of many types. Some pains are felt by heart like William Sheksppeare has written in 'As you like it' "Blow-blow thou winter wind, thou biteis not so sharp as a man's ingratitude"

But here, in this book, I have discussed only about body pains. Pains of different joints, abdomen, menstrual colic, angina etc. are discussed and their probable treatment and management is also described.

This book is useful for all age groups. Illustrations of accupressure treatment are also given, which is supposed to be good supportive therapy for body pains. There are two separate chapters of homoeopathic treatment and a chapter on ayurvedic treatment too alongwith diet plan and home remedies. Initially I have discussed the body parts and their function for the knowledge of readers.

If you have any querry, you can write to me with a reply envelope. If you want to come to my place, first fix an appointment and please do not come without appointment.

With thanks and regards.

**—Dr. Rajeev Sharma**

Srijan - Aarogya Jyoti®

Palm-11/03, Shipra Sun City

Indirapuram, Ghaziabad(U.P.)

Phone- 0120-3020206

E-mail: sharmarajeev108@rediffmail.com

rrajeev@newkamasutra.com

# CONTENTS

## Some Other Body Pains

# 1

# Human Body System

There are eight basic systems of the human body (i) Skeletal System (ii) Muscular System (iii) Circulatory System (iv) Nervous System (v) Respiratory System (vi) Digestive system (vii) Excretory System (viii) Reproductive System. I will discuss these one by one.

## The Skeletal System

The bony skeleton supporting the human body is constructed to strengthen the muscles which produce movement in the body to give shape. The forelimbs of the human body are supported by bones forming a shoulder girdle and similarly the leg bones are connected to others forming a pelvic girdle. Ribs connected to the backbone (including those connected to the breast bone) serve to protect certain internal organs, including the heart and the lungs. Man's structural superiority over other animals is due to the straight femur or thigh bone and the erect poise of the head.

The above features enable the man to' walk in an erect position so that his hands are tree to perform other functions. These structural advantages and the formation of his skull and lower jaw are responsible for an increase in brain power and intelligence in man, as compared with the other animals.

The human system consists of 206 bones of various sizes. The bones are composed of cells, which are softer in early childhood than in adult life. Where bones meet there is a joint which may simply be an immovable joint as in the bones of the skull or may be movable joint as that of the knee. The movable joints are necessary for the motion of human body.

## Muscular System

Muscles are attached to the bones and consist of bundles of fleshly fibres, capable of contraction or shortening. When required such contractions help the various limbs of the body to move. The muscles are of two kinds namely the voluntary muscles whose movements are controlled by human will and the involuntary muscles which perform their function without any conscious effort of the will. These include the heart, the muscles of the stomach and those of the intestines. Their movements are rhythmic and we are not conscious of their action.

## The Circulatory System

This system comprises the blood and heart and their functions. The blood is continuously propelled by the contraction of the heart and is derived into the arteries. The arteries are elastic tubes which by their recoil aid the distribution of the blood to all parts.

The blood is a clear fluid comprising innumberable solid bodies called corpuscles. The corpuscles are of two kinds -red and white- and are cellular shaped. The red corpuscles carry haemoglobin which constitutes protein and a little iron.

When combined with oxygen haemoglobin forms a bright red substance. The white corpuscles are living organisms, small jelly like creatures each with a nucleus. They are of great importance as they eat up the disease germs that enter the body. They are capable of independent movement in the blood stream and within the tissue and can swallow up dead bacteria and foreign particles.

The main functions of blood are the following:

- It carries oxygen to every part of the body that requires it.
- It carries impurities from all parts of the body to the excretory organs namely the lungs, the kidneys and the skin.
- It carries food from the digestive system to all tissues.
- It carries heat to all parts of the body.

The heart is a hollow, muscular and somewhat conical four chambered force pump enclosed in a fibrous bag. It is situated in the chest between the lungs and weigh from 10 to 12 ounces. The heart is divided into two parts by a wall running from top to bottom with no direct connection between the parts. These parts are themselves divided into parts, upper and lower but have valves between them. The upper portions are called Auricles and the lower ones Ventricles.

When the blood reaches the tissues it loses all its oxygen and is loaded with waste materials especially carbon dioxide from the tissues. The impure blood reaches the heart by means of capillaries and veins. With the beat of the heart, it enters into the Right Auricle and then to the Right Ventricle from where it is taken by the pulmonary Artery to the lungs. In the lungs capillaries, the blood comes into contact with oxygen and is purified (oxygenated). The purified blood is now brought back to heart by means of Pulmonary Vein. It now enters the left Auricle and when auricles are contracted during the heart beat, the blood passes to the left Ventricle and then commences its journey again to all parts of the body. Thus with the contraction of right and left auricles, the venous blood from the body ana aerated (oxygenated) blood from the lungs is pumped into their respective ventricles. And when the right and left ventricles contract, venous blood is pumped into the lungs and the aerated blood into the main vessels. These rhythmic contractions and dilations followed by an equivalent pause are called pulse or heart beat.

## The Nervous System

It is the most important system as it commands rest of the body what to do and how to work together. While the central nervous system resides in the skull and the spine, the nerves are spread all over the body. The nervous system of a man is a network pervading the whole body, having two way connection with the central control and enabling the individual to give a coordinated response to any stimulus from outside. Thus nerves that carry the messages to the muscles with orders to perform a particular action are called Motor Nerves.

The brain is the chief centre of the nervous system and is contained within the skull. The brain susbstance consists of grey and white matter. The grey matter forming a thin, superficial layer (cortex). It consists of three parts: (a) the cerebrum or bigger brain, which governs our consciousness, thought, emotions, will, sight, hearing, sensation of pain and memory through the grey matter, (b) the cerebellum or the smaller brain is connected with the coordination of the actions, nervous and muscular, by which the movement of the body are carried on, (c) Medulla Oblongata houses the centre of nervous tissue connected with reflex action consisting of movements that take place automatically, such as breathing or walking.

The spinal cord consist mostly of nerves. This is like a continuation of the medulla and runs down the back, surrounded by the bony arch of the spinal column. This organ is capable of making simple decisions, called the reflex action.

## The Respiratory System

This system comprises lungs and the passages leading to them.

The purpose of respiration (breathing) is the entry and exit of air to and from the lungs. The object of breathing is to bring oxygen of the air into contact with the blood with the purpose of (a) giving some oxygen to the blood and (b) taking out waste products from the blood.

The air, in going to the lungs, has to go through various passages. They are nose or mouth, and the larynx or voice box.

We breathe through nose or through mouth. There are two passages leading downwards from nose and mouth into the body one takes food and water to the stomach and the other takes air to the lungs.

Larynx or voice box is commonly known as "Adam's Apple" and can easily be felt in the throat. It is a cavity (inthroat) holding vocal cords. Vibration of cords produces vocal sounds. The air passes from the voice box to the lungs by means of wind pipe which is about four inches long and one inch wide. The wind pipe at the lower end, is divided into two branches that go to the lungs.

The functioning of the lungs has already been described while discussing the Excretory System. The functioning of lungs as the respiratory organ is slightly more complicated. In the lungs, the air gets very close to the blood, that comes from the whole body through heart. The impure blood, dark red in colour, has too much carbon dioxide in it. This blood comes from the tissues, which have taken the oxygen from it but have loaded it with carbon dioxide. In the tissues, oxygen is used every minute to bum up the food material, resulting in production of considerable quantity of carbon dioxide. The lung's function is to reverse this state of affairs, i.e. restoring its oxygen quota and expelling the excess carbondioxide. Thus the venous blood (the impure blood) is rendered arterial (bright red in colour) in its passage through the lung capillaries. It goes back to the heart and is ready to do its work again. The fresh oxygen, taken by the blood all over the body, is picked up again by its muscles which need it for their normal functioning.

## Digestive System

The food that we take comprises proteins, sugars and starches, vitamins, salts, fats and oils. Only a part of these substances is useful to the body and the rest, which is indigestible, must be get rid of. The foot is broken up by the teeth and after getting mixed with saliva, it is swallowed. Saliva is an alkaline fluid which is also common to the air passage at this level. It then passes into the gullet. Like stomach and intestines, the gullet is a muscular organ and can force the food along if necessary. With the help of the muscle, a man can drink even if he is standing on his head. About nine inches long, the gullet ends in the stomach. It is here that the second stage of digestion takes place.

From this position the food reaches stomach which is a hollow muscular organ lined by a glandular mucus membrane which secretes the gastric juice containing hydrochloric acid, salts, pepsin and water. The stomach mixes the food well by moving it round and round. At one stage the proteins are changed to a form in which they can pass through the stomach well and be absorbed, at once, ready to nourish the body.

Starches and proteins are now acted upon, though not digested completely. Fat and oil are broken up and oil is set free. In the stomach, digestion may take two to three hours. The food then goes to small intestine which is a long tube which, when uncoiled, may measure about one feet. Here, we have to consider the action of three different digestive juices, e.g., the pancreatic juice, the bile generated by the liver and the intestinal juice, which is the secretion of the small glands of the bowel lining. Food passes through the intestine and finally nutrients are absorbed and carried into the blood. The bile and the pancreatic juices are produced by the liver and pancreas respectively.

Liver is the largest organ in the body, which is situated just underneath the diaphragm rather on the right side. Its weight is about three to four pounds. There are fine tubes in the liver called bile ducts into which the cells of the liver secrete vile, and the bile ducts join together and form Hepatic duct which carries the bile to the duodenum (also known as first part of small intestine).

Bile is a yellow fluid, containing mucus, water and some salts (called bile salts). It acts on the fats and oils and breaks them up into very small particles.

Liver is also a storehouse for sugar which it puts in the blood, when it is required by the body. About seven inches long, there is another large gland reddish in colour and known as Pancrea,s. It lies behind the stomach, and tube from it called the Pancreatic duct enters the intestine near where the bile duct enters. The pancreatic juices act on the protein the starches and the fats.

The intestine is an organ of digestion as well as of absorption. The food, now digested, can pass through the walls of the intestine and is taken into the blood. It is then distributed allover the body. Food remains in the small intestine for about 12 hours and is slowly passed on towards the large intestine.

The large intestine is a 6 feet long tube. It is little concerned with the digestion or absorption of food, for more of this has already been done. Food remains here from 24 to 36 hours. Due to loss of water, the material in the large intestine now hardens as it reaches the rectum. Finally, the ingestible remnant is turned out.

## The Excretory System

It comprises the kidney, skin, lungs and bowels. The system is designed to help get rid of the waste matter in the body when all juices have been extracted from the digestive food. There are two kidneys, situated one on each side of the backbone in the small portion of the back or loin. It has the renal artery which brings blood to it and the renal vein which takes it away. In addition, there are the usual nerves, the lymphatic vessels and the ureter, the tube that takes urine from the kidney to the bladder which is the reservoir for urine.

Urine, a pale yellow fluid, carrying the waste nitrogen from our protein foods, and also mineral salts, secreted into the two kidneys. The kidney may be regarded as a pair of filters, through which about 2 pints of blood circulates every minute. In fact, the whole blood in the body passes down to the kidneys in five to six minutes. Urine is propelled down along the ureters from the kidneys to the bladder by successive veins of contraction in the muscular walls of these channels.

The bladder is an elastic membrance serving as temporary reservoir for urine, secreted by the kidneys. The normal adult capacity is about 1 pint. The urine is discharged into the bladder in intermittent jets every 20 seconds or so. The outlet below the bladder is normally closed by a tight ring of muscle called sphincter. In emptying, the bladder contracts and the sphincter relaxes to allow efflux of urine.

Another important agent for excretion of the waste material from the body is skin. It has two layers, the top one called the epidermis and dermis or true skin below the epidemics.

The latter is richly supplied with blood vessels. The skin is designed to:

- protect the body;

- act as an organ of excretion by means of sweat glands. It thus helps to regulate the temperature of the body and;
- to give the sense of touch.

The skin has hair and sense organs. The latter are little lumps in the dermis which are nerve ending. They report to the nervous system when anything comes into their contant. The skin also has two kinds of glands, the Sebaceous glands, which secrete an oily substance serving as lubricant to the skin and the sweat glands which make the skin as an excretory organ. The function of the latter is to take up sweat from the blood and pour it out on the skin. Though mostly water, the sweat contains, salts, fats and tiny bits of skin.

Bowels are the intestines, both large and small, which serve to complete the digestion of food and to allow its absorption into the blood stream. The useless or undigested food remains are gradually moved onwards and are hardened in the large intestine wherefrom they are ready to be thrown out. The failure of the bowel function is called constipation.

Lumps comprise two elastic spongy masses, almost filling the chest cavity. These are import agents to cleanse the system of impurity. Lungs throw off carbon dioxide, water (in the shape of vapour) and also some organic matter.

They are, therefore, organs of excretion in addition to being the organs of respiration

## Reproductive System

Sex is an act preformed emotionaly and physically sex organs play an important role. Hope is the description of sex organs-

## Male Organs

The sex organs of a male are quite complicated form of a reproductive system. They produce semen store it and release into the woman's vagina at the time of ejaculation. Procreation, therefore, is the result of the union of the sperm cell and the ovum.

## Testes

The male organs comprise of the two testes of testicles hung side by side in a sac called the scrotum, behind the penis in its relaxed state. The testes are oval in shape and about an inch long and inch wide, have two different functions. These are made up of a series of lobes composed of minute tubules in which the sperm cells the spermatozoa are formed and liberated. The internal secretion of sex hormones which create sex impulses and cause the essential male characteristics in the individual and play its role with the other secretory glands in the body in sustaining the normal functioning of the body, are achieved by it. In case this function is impaired before puberty, the development of the individual becomes seriously altered in form, temperament and impulses. Since it is directly absorbed into the blood, these secretions are termed as internal secretions.

In the seminal discharge the male sperms formed in the testes are the vital elements because these sperms have the power of fertilising the egg of the woman to conceive a new life. These highly vitalized cells consist of a head, neck and long tail. It is in this head that the nucleus is contained which transmit the hereditary characteristics of the individual. Having the power of independent motion these sperms propel themselves in the liquid secretion in which it floats, it requires an hour or more for the sperm to reach the cavity of the uterus and a few hours to gain the oviduct or the tube where it fertilises an ovum (egg). When the released female egg encounters one male sperm or spermatozoon it penetrates the cell wall of the egg in an complex series of rearrangement of both cells, known as fertilisation. Though, in single male organism about 200 to 500 million sperms are discharged, only one is able to reach the walls of the cell. The remaining cells are cast out along with the other residues of the physiological process. The spermatozoa are being slowly formed and released in the testicles all the time.

## Epididymis and Vas Deferens

Each of the cluste of convoluted tubes in the lobes of the testes in which the sperm cells are formed merges into a single tube and the resulting mass of tubes in turn forms a complex network which constitutes a large annexe to the body of the testes. It is known as epididymis. The network of the tubes of epididymis unite in turn to form the seminal duct or vas defrens. From the epididymis each seminal duct passes upwards in the scrotal sac and enters the pelvis cavity where it continues its upward course, then curves forward and downward to enter the urethra which conducts the urine from the bladder.

## Seminal Vesides

The vas two in number, issuing from each testes takes a round of the bladder and then empty into the seminal vesicles. These vesicles are two small pouches, situated just behind the urinary bladder. The function of seminal vesicles is to store the semen and secrete a gelatinus substance which by mixing with the sperm thickens the semen and increases its volume. The secretion, the sperm thickens the semen and increases its volume. The secretion also provides nourishment and strength to sperms.

Since these testes and seminal vesicles are always secreting and manufacturing semen, sometimes the vesicles are filled to capacity and the nature empties them in the form of nocturnal emissions as is in the process orgasm.

The phenomenon is usually accompanied by erotic dreams and pleasurable sex feelings of an orgasm.

It is a mistaken belief of old theories that nocturnal emissions or wet dreams are a sign of weaknes. These are natural, harmless occurrence to be expected in most normal men., particularly between the ages of fourteen and thirty-five. There is nothing to worry about. Untold mental torture and unnecessary expense has been caused to millions of men through the misrepresentation of quacks and fear of men in these matters.

Seminal emissions vary greatly in frequency of occurrence between different men and in the same man at different times. Within the normal the frequency may range between once a month to several times a week . Many factors, physical, mental and temperamental- are responsible for it. There are some young men who rarely or never experience nocturnal emissions. Though the occurrence of emissions are natural, their absence does not necessarily indicate any abnormality. It is quite possible in their case that the contents naturally ooze out in the ducts aided by bowel movements, to be thrown out with the urine from the bladder.

Nocturnal emissions generally occur when a man sleeps on his back. The reason being that in this position the weight of the partly filled or full bladder resting upon the vesicles increases the irritation to set of the reflexes ejuculating semen. To avoid this, heavy food should not be taken before going to bed and constipation should not be allowed.

## Prostate Gland

It is shaped like a horse chest nut . Surrounding the neck of the bladder and the junction of the urinary and spermatic ducts, into which juncture the prostate empties its contents through some thirty outlets. The prostrate secretion is also added to the semen before it is ejaculated in the vagina. thus semen is a combined product of all these glands. Each of these glands imparts to the semen its many peculiar characteristics. The prostate is also a sexual gland, which is situated below the urinary bladder. During coital climax, the prostate cntracts and mixes its own secretion in the semen. To sustain sexual vigour and strength, it is considered necessary that the prostate functions properly. The prostate secretes a thin milky, alkaline fluid the function of which is similar to the products of the vesicles. The alkalinity serves to protect the spermatozoa against acidity arising from the urine. The acidity damages the vitality of the sperm cells.

## Urethra

A small duct called urethra runs through the centre of the penis down to its glands from the urinary bladder. This duct serves the double purpose it empties the urine from the bladder and ejaculates the semen from the seminal vesicles. thus, urethra is connected with both the systems of seminal discharge and urine elimination. The urethra in penis discharges both semen and urine but sex mechanism of male body is such that both the actions cannot take place together. During seminal discharge a special valve automatically shuts off the urine.

## Penis

A child's penis is small which grows long with the other organ of the body after the onset of puberty. Penis through which the bladder is emptied and the sperm is discharged during intercourse, is normally three to four inches long and in normal flaccid state about one and a quarter to tow inches in diameter. When a man is sexually aroused his penis grows erect and organ measures about one and a half inches in diameter and five and half to six and a half inches in length along its upper side. It is made up in part of spongy tissue which becomes gorged with blood, making the organ hard and rigid , In excited state it stands out an angle from the body to confirm in general to the normal vagina angle of the woman . The erection is essential in order to achieve the penetration of the vagina. In response to mechanical or psychic stimulation, the erction is achieved through a nervous mechanism which causes a rush of blood into the organ and at the same time greatly restricts its flow thus, causing rigid distention of the penis, Like the size, the shape also varies from man to man. Penis is the male copulating organ which conducts the semen into vagina. There is no correlation betwen the size of a penis and a man's sexual strength and capacity. The erect size also does not make much difference because vagina has such an elastic cavity to accommodate any size of penis. The most sensitive nerve ending in a vagina is the clitoris which can always be reached by any penis howsoever it be small.

## Glans Penis

The foremost end of the penis round like a knob is called glans penis. It is slight thicker than the rest of the shaft. In the flaccid state of the penis the head or glans penis is partly or wholly by a loose layer of the skin, in the uncirumcised, called the prepuce of foreskin. This is retract for the purpose of cleaning and it becomes natural retracted after entry in coitus. The surface of the foreskin is somewhat mucus owing to the glans which secrete a substance called smegna. It is an irritating secretion and should be regularly cleaned, otherwise it makes the forepart of the penis become chessy in appearance by breeding germs. It should be daily washed with soap. The glans penis has the most sensitive nerve endings. A slight soft touch is enough to excite a man and to make the penis erect. It is mainly the glans penis on which a little rubbing whether by hand or by vaginal contact sends the sex waves in the entire body, culminating in orgasm or ejaculation.

## Erection and Ejaculation

As also referred to earlier, the effect of the sexual arousal in man is physically manifest in the erection of the penis. A direct and gently stimulation of the penis almost always causes erection. This is borne out of reflex action and may occur in sleep. Erection may be caused without any rubbing of the penis, just by erotic thoughts or dreams it goes erect. In the early morning it may be aroused becuse of the urge to urinate. Most such erections terminate without any discharge.

Ejaculation is the culmination of sexual stimulation in man. Having entered the vagina, the most sensitive nerve endings of which the penis is made up, become tense and excited on account of the friction against the walls of vagina, the cozy heat it may experience further fanned by the secretion of the fluid in the vagina. To and fro movements of the penis add on the arousal. The tension gets higher and higher till it reaches the climax and the release of the seminal fluids is known as ejaculation. The basic difference between the sex mechanism of the man and the woman is, in man the climax and ejaculation or orgasm take place simultaneously while in woman these are two different states. At the time of the climaxic height orgasm the seminal discharge takes place through the penis in a number of spurts.The number of the spurts varies from 4 to 20 just as the first menses indicates the onset of puberty in a girl,the first ejaculation marks the boy's entrance into adolescence.

## Female Organs

The female organs are more complicated because they are confined in the body and not openly visible. Because of the apparent invisibility most of the girls are unaware about their internal sex organs. Hence , it is all the more necessary that full knowledge about the female organs structure and their function be discussed in full details.

## Vulva

The two visibly fleshy folds, covered with hair are the outer lips or labia majora. When parted they reveal two smaller or inner lips of labia. The insides of the inner labia are covered with mucous membrnae. The inner lips or labia are one of the several sexual sensation centres. In sexual intercourse these labia remain constantly massaged by the rubbing of penis. In some women the inner lips protrude somewhat. The inner lips meet their upper ends which when separated look like the form of wish bone of a hen.

The principle of the sex feeling, the clitoris is situated just above the junction of the inner lips. The clitoris looks like a mini penis having erectile tissue and a head and foreskin similar to the penis of the man. It is covered from above by a hood of skin. The clitoris is made up of highly sensitive nerves which respond very well to sexual stimulation. It is from this centre that the sexual feeling begins and permeates in the entire body through vulva and vagina. When erect the clitoris looks like the size of or shape of small bean. about an inch below the clitoris a small opening of the tube called urethra. Its duct conducts the urine from the bladder. The urethra has only the urinary function and no sexual function.

The muscous membrane above the clitoris , like the penis of a man, is covered with glands which secrete smegna. Owing to the structure, cleanliness in the woman is somewhat more difficult than it is in the man.

It is not hygeinically necessary to keep it clean but also for this reason that it emits smell which tend to inhbit sexual desire in the man.

## Hymen

Just below the urinary passage is the entrance to vagina. In the normal virgin girl this opening remains partially close by a thin membrane called the hymen. Though it appears in different shapes but normally it looks like a crescent in shape appearing the forward extension of the black walls of the vagina. In many cases during the first intercourse when the hymen is ruptured there may be slight bleeding and pain. But this should not cause any alarm. It is a false notion which the orthodox still maintain that the hymen is the symbol of virginity. A nicked or stretched or tattered hymen does not mean that the body has been penetrated into. It could be ruptured on account of many a jerks or falls that a young girl might have experienced. Many girls may not have much of it or others may lose it in doing some kind of vigorous job. sometimes the insertion of a finger into the vagina may prove too hard for any hymen. Occasionally a hymen is so tough that it remains intact even after several sessions of sexual intercourses. It all depends on the kind of hymen a girl is born with. Generally during the first coitus, the penis tear it till hardly a few shreds mark it former presence. At times in certain cases it was found to be so flexible that instead of breaking into pieces by the penile thrust, it merely bends and allows the penis to glide over it. It may in certain cases remain there even after delivering a child. In some cases the surgeon's aid is obtained to slit open the membrane. But the bleeding and discomfort, when they occur are not of sufficient consequence to warrant fear on the part of the woman. This is psychologically important because this fear powerfully inhibits her sexusl responses and the function of the lubricating glands, leaving the parts dry. This increases the probability of discomfort and bleeding and diminishes the possibility of experiencing any sex pleasure at the first coitus.

## Vagina

It is a tube or canal extending from vulva to the neck of the uterus. It is three and half to 4 inches in length in its normal relaxed position. It is here that the penis in intercourse is sheathed with its elastic walls. It receives the seminal discharge and allows the sperm to travel forward towards the womb in search of the ovum. It is through this tube that a child passes to the outside world during pregnancy the vagina and its outlet becomes capable to great expansion, permitting the passage of the child from the womb without injury in many cases. In most instances, however more or less laceration of the muscular structure controlling the opening and of the vagina itself occurs. It should be vitally important that such tears receive prompt surgical attention. The use and control of the muslces about the vaginal opening of the enire pelvic floor are necessary to woman's most effective participation in coitus. The relaxed condition and the loss of muscular control which results from the failure to repair perineal and vaginal teras may result in greatly diminishing sexual satisfaction in coitus for both partners and may render it impossible for the woman to achieve orgasm at all. The flexible walls of the vagina are lined moist and clean. It has a great relaxing and contracting power. It is because of this reason that the vagins, besides being made up of flexible walls, is able to accommodate must larger penis not with standing its small cavity.

## Womb or Uterus

It is pear shaped organ of heavy muscular walls. The virgin uterus measures about two inches wide. Its elastic muscles expand considerably during pregnancy with the growth of the baby. Its upper part is connected with ovaries by two ducts called fallopian tubes. The organ is supported in the pelvis by strong ligaments, its position is at right angles to the vagina, the upper, heavy end being directed forward towards the front of the pelvis. The small end opens into the vagina and closes its upper end. After childbirth the organ gradually retracts to its normal size. The organ has powerful muscles to help push the baby out through the vagina. During pregnancy, the uterus retains and supplies nourishment to the growing baby till the delivery.

## Fallopian Tubes and Ovaries

The upper end of the uterus as referred earlier are joined by the fallopian tubes, each about five and half inches long. Which extend right and left to the ovaries. The function of the fallopian tube is to conduct ovum from the ovaries to the uterus. This is achieved through contractile action of the tubes finger like fringes called fimbria. The sweeping motion of fimbria is in one direction, which helps the egg cells in moving towards uterus. In most cases, the fertilisation of an egg cell or ovum takes place during its journey through the fallopian tube . The process of passing an egg cell through the tube is called ovulation. The fertilised egg is then moved down the tube towards the womb.

The ovaries can be compared likened to the testes of the male. They produce the female reproductive cells, the ova (eggs) and internal secretions. Situated at the outer ends of the tubes, one on each side of the uterus, an ovary is about the size and shape of a large almond in the shell. though they are comparable to the testes in their function, the hormone function of the ovaries is apparently more complex than that of the testes of the male. In addition to the internal secretion which governs development of the specific female character and help to sustain the normal functioning of the individual as an organism, the ovaries elaborate other chemical substances which control the reproductive functions. If the ovaries are removed before puberty the development of the individual gets drastically altered. Even after marriage, if ovary is removed for any reason, there could be certain changes felt physically and mentally.

When a girl is born, here ovaries already contain these egg cells or ova in tens of thousands. But then these are not mature. With the onset of puberty the ovaries start their work of maturing ovum. During the life time of woman about 400 --500 of egg cells mature. From the time of puberty till menopause, every month a mature egg is produced by one of the ovaries. The mature egg cell passes through the fallopian tube towards the uterus. If an egg is fertilised it starts growing before it enters the velvety lined uterus which nourishes the egg well. If the egg is not fertilised it remains alive for about 20-44 hours after entering the tube and then it disintegrates and gets absorbed into the body. In that case soft and velvety lining of uterus is not required, the blood and the blood vessels forming the protective lining are cast out through vagina.

## Menstruation

When the egg cell is not fertilised, the monthly preparation by the womb to receive a fertilised egg cell gove a waste and the debris is cast out the whole process is known as menstruation. Menstruation generally continues for three to five days but even longer in few cases. While it is a normal physiological function, not to be regarded as a 'sickness' or being 'unwell' in several cases the general let down and the re ad justments of the entire organism do involve nervous tensions and in many cases a variety of aches and pains for which due allowance is to be made in the social and personal circle of the individual. It should be clearly understood that a girl or woman during the periods, should not be considered an ' untouchable' . As a matter of fact, the underlying reason of this belief was sympathetic- that in a period of menstruation, a girl or a lady might feel weak so she should be given full rest- which has been mistakenly converted into a hygienic one. But now a days not educated girl or woman adhere to these obscurantic norms and treat the period days like any other day in their life. May be, because of better facilities to contain this blood into the sanitary napkins, the modern woman does not make it a show of it. It is not physically but emotionally a woman might feel disturbed during this period, for which she should be shown due consideration.

### Breasts

Though the breasts do not strictly come under the categories of the organs we are discussing, they are being induced because of their special significance in manifestation of the sexual arousal of a woman. Specially their breasts' nipples signify as one of the most erogenous zones on woman's body. Squeezing, sucking, touching, caressing of the breasts, particularly the nipples give rise to strong and most favourable sexual desires. The sexologists say that in the initial stages of married life a woman derives more pleasure from any such stimulation of her breast than the actual coitus. Nipples, like clitoris have erectile tissues and very sensitive nerve endings. The tissues become firm and erect during erotic stimulation.

It is for this reason that breasts or mammary glands are two very important sexual organs, whose development is dependent on the secretion of certain hormones of the female sex. Though, the breasts have their primary function in feeding a new born child there importance as an erotic and sensitive zone permeating with desire to mate has great significance in sexual relationship. Although their sizes vary from puberty to maturity and they grow large during pregnancy. The sexual undertones of this organ has influenced the loving onlookers most. an ideally formed breast has always been the most beautiful female symbol or characteristic. The another most important function of breasts is to feed child after delivery.

# 2

# ARTHRITIS PAIN AND IT'S RELIEF

The pain of arthritis may come from different sources. These may include inflammation of the synovial membrane (tissue that lines the joints), the tendons, or the ligaments; muscle strain; and fatigue. A combination of these factors contributes to the intensity of the pain.

The pain of arthritis varies greatly from person to person, for reasons that doctors do not yet understand completely. Factors that contribute to the pain include swelling within the joint, the amount of heat or redness present, or damage that has occured within the joint. In addition, activities affect pain differently so that some patients not pain in their joints after first getting out of bed in the morning whereas others develop pain after prolonged use of the joint. Each individual has a different threshold and tolerance for pain, often affected by both physical and emotional factors. These can include depression, anxiety, and even hypersensitivity at the affected sites due to inflammation and .tissue injury. This increased sensitivity appears to affect the amount of pain perceived by the individual.

## Measuring Arthritis Pain?

Pain is a private, unique experience that cannot be seen. The most common way to measure pain is for the doctor to ask you, the patient, about your problems. For example, the doctor may ask you to describe the level of pain you feel on a scale of 1 to 10. You may use words like aching, burning, stinging, or throbbing. These words will give the doctor a clearer picture of the pain you are experiencing. Since doctors rely on your description of pain to help guide treatment, you may want to keep a pain diary to record your pain sensations. On a daily basis, you can describe the situations that cause or alter the intensity of your pain, the sensations and severity of your pain, and your reactions to the pain. For example:

"On Sunday night, sharp pains in my knees produced by housework interfered with my sleep; on Monday morning, because of the pain, I had a hard time getting out bed. However, I coped with the pain by taking my medication and applying ice to my knees."

The diary will give the doctor some insight into your pain and may play a critical role in the management of your disease.

What will Happen when You First Visit a Doctor for your Arthritis Pain?

The doctor will usually do the following:

- Take your medical history and ask questions such as: How long have you had this problem? How intense is the pain? How often does it occur? What causes it to get worse? What causes it to get better?
- Review the medications you are using
- Conduct a physical examination
- Take blood and/or urine samples and request necessary laboratory work
- Ask you to get X-rays taken or undergo other imaging procedures such as a CAT scan (computerized axial tomography) or MRI (magnetic resonance imaging).

Once the doctor has done these things and reviewed the results of any tests or procedures, he or she will discuss the findings with you and design a comprehensive management approach for the pain caused by your osteoarthritis or rheumatoid arthritis.

## Who Can Treat Arthritis Pain?

A number of different specialists may be involved in the care of an arthritis patient often a team approach is used. The team may include doctors who treat people with arthritis (rheumatologists), surgeons (orthopaedists), and physical and occupational therapists. Their goal is to treat all aspects of arthritis pain and help you learn to manage your pain. The physician, other health care professionals, and you, the patient, all play an active role in the management of arthritis pain.

## How is Arthritis Pain Treated?

There is no single treatment that applies to all people with arthritis, but rather the doctor will develop a management plan designed to minimize your specific pain and improve the function of your joints. A number of treatments can provide short-term pain relief.

## Short-Term Relief

- Medications: Because people with osteoarthritis have very little inflammation, pain relievers such as acetaminophen (Tylenol) may be effective. Patients with rheumatoid arthritis generally have pain caused by inflammation and often benefit from aspirin or other nonsteroidal antiinflammatory drugs (NSAIDs) such as ibuprofen.
- Heat and cold: The decision to use either heat or cold for arthritis pain depends on the type of arthritis and should be discussed with your doctor or physical therapist. Moist heat, such as a warm bath or shower, or dry heat, such as a heating pad, placed on the painful area of the joint for about

15 minutes may relieve the pain. An ice pack (or a bag of frozen vegetables) wrapped in a towel and placed on the sore area for about 15 minutes may help to reduce swelling and stop the pain. If you have poor circulation, do not use cold packs.

- Joint Protection: Using a splint or a brace to allow joints to rest and protect them from injury can be helpful. Your physician or physical therapist can make recommendations.
- Transcutaneous electrical nerve stimulotion (TENS): A small TENS device that directs mild electric pulses to nerve endings that lie beneath the skin in the painful area may relieve some arthritis pain. TENS seems to work by blocking pain messages to the brain and by modifying pain perception.
- Massage: In this pain-relief approach, a massage therapist will lightly stroke and/or knead the painful muscle. This may increase blood flow and bring warmth to a stressed area. However, arthritis-stressed joints are very sensitive so the therapist must be very familiar with the problems of the disease.
- Acupuncture: This procedure should only be done by a licensed acupuncture therapist. In acupuncture, thin needles are inserted at specific points in the body. Scientists think that this stimulates the release of natural, pain-relieving chemicals produced by the brain or the nervous system.

Osteoarthritis and rheumatoid arthritis are chronic diseases that may last a lifetime. Learning how to manage your pain over the long term is an important factor in controlling the disease and maintaining a good quality of life. Following are some sources of long- term pain relief.

## Long-Term Relief

- Medications:

Nonsteroidal anti-inflammatory drugs (NSAIDs): These are a class of drugs including aspirin and ibuprofen that are used to reduce pain and inflammation and may be used for both short-term and long-term relief in people with osteoarthritis and rheumatoid arthritis.

Disease-modifying anti-rheumatic drugs (DMARDS): These are drugs used to treat people with rheumatoid arthritis who have not responded to NSAIDs. Some of these include methotrexate, hydroxychloroquine. penicillamine and gold injections. These drugs are thought to influence and correct abnormalities of the immune system responsible for a disease like rheumatoid arthritis. Treatment with these medications requires careful monitoring by the physician to avoid side effects.

Corticosteroids: These are hormones that are very effective in treating arthritis. Corticosteroids can be taken by mouth or given by injection. Prednisone is the corticosteroid most often given by mouth to reduce the inflammation of rheumatoid arthritis. In both rheumatoid arthritis and osteoarthritis, the doctor also may inject a corticosteroid into the affected joint to stop pain. Because frequent injections may cause damage to the cartilage they should only be done once or twice a year.

- Weight reduction: Excess pounds put extra stress on weight-bearing joints such as the knees or hips. Studies have shown that overweight women who lost an average of 11 pounds substantially reduced the development of osteoarthritis in their knees. In addition, if osteoarthritis has already affected one knee, weight reduction will reduce the chance of it occurring in the other knee.
- Exercise: Swimming, walking, low-impact aerobic exercise and range-of- motion exercises may reduce

joint pain and stiffness. In addition, stretching exercises are helpful. A physical therapist can help plan an exercise program that will give you the most benefit.

- Surgery: In select patients with arthritis, surgery may be necessary. The surgeon may perform an operation to remove the synovium (synovectomy), realign the joint (osteotomy). or in advanced cases replace the damaged joint with an artificial one. Total joint replacement has provided not only dramatic relief from pain but also improvement in motion for many people with arthritis.

## How Can You Cope with Arthritis Pain?

The long-term goal of pain management is to help you cope with a chronic, often disabling disease. You may be caught in a cycle of pain, depression and stress. To break out of this cycle, you need to be an active participant with the doctor and other health care professionals in managing your pain. This may include physical therapy, cognitive-behavioral therapy, occupational therapy, biofeedback, relaxation techniques (for example, deep breathing and meditation), and family counseling therapy.

Another technique is to substitute distraction for pain. Focus your attention on things that you enjoy. Imagine a peaceful setting and wonderful physicol sensations. Thinking about something that is enjoyable can help you relax and become less stressed. Find something that will make you laugh, a cartoon, a funny movie, or even a new joke. Try to put some joy back into your life. Even a small change in your mental image may break the pain cycle and provide relief.

## What Research is Being Conducted On Arthritis Pain?

Recent NIAMS studies show that levels of several neuropeptides (compounds produced by cells of the nervous system), such as substance P, are increased in arthritic joints. Substance P is involved in the transmission of pain signals via the nervous system. At the University of Missouri, researchers are studying effects of substance P in the spines of animals with chronic arthritis. Findings from this study may be used to develop specific drugs for chronic pain such as that associated with arthritis.

Researchers are also studying the human knee and analyzing how injury in one joint may affect other joints. In addition, they are analysing the effect of pain and analgesics on gait (walking) and comparing pain and gait before and after surgical treatment of knee osteoarthritis.

3

# KNEE PAIN—CAUSES AND TYPES

Knee pain may subside on its own within a few days or persist for weeks or months. When the pain subsides within a few days, it is often due to minor problems such as a 'sprain'. When the knee pain persists for longer time, its causes can:

1. Pain due to injury to the knee;
2. Pain due to conditions not associated with injury.

Knee Sprain—causes and symptoms

- Common in day-to-day activities due to minor twisting or bending.
- Pain in subsides within a few days to a week.
- Injury to semilunar cartilages.
- Caused when the knee is twisted or while landing on the knee suddenly.
- Pain may not subside within a few days.
- May give a feeling of something "getting stuck" or "loose" inside the knee.
- Knee may be locked in one position.

Injury to ligaments of the knee–causes and symptoms

- Front middle ligament often injured in sports when a sudden load comes on the knee or while jumping from a height.
- May also be due to forced twisting of the knee.
- May result in a 'sound' of something breaking inside the knee when the ligaments are injured.
- Rapid swelling of the knee because the blood fills the joint.

## Fractures and Dislocations–causes and symptoms

Fractures may involve

- lower end of the thigh bone
- upper end of the bone or
- the kneecap
- Acute pain with immediate swelling
- Knee cap dislocation is common in adolescents
- Recurrent dislocation of knee cap is common

## Overuse Injuries–causes and symptoms

- Common in sports persons and military recruits due to excessive demand on the joint.
- Pain occurs when adolescents or fresh military recruits undertake new or excessive physical activity.
- Injuries are usually due to a mild problem in the 'design' of the knee.
- Overuse injuries usually cause pain under stressful situation.

Injury to the knee is common in sports, accidents and sometimes day-to-day activities. It is a common cause of knee pain in younger people. There are several types or injuries to the knee joint such as tears in the meniscus, ligaments, etc. which are collectively known as 'Internal Derangement of the Knee' (or 'I.D.K.'). Sometimes it is difficult to diagnose the exact type of derangement, and therefore some people consider I.D.K. as synonymous with 'I Don't know'.

Some causes of knee pain are not associated with injury and often cause pain in other joints also. The main group of diseases in this category is **arthritis.** The word "arthiritis" does not mean one disease–it means pain and swelling of a joint. There could be many reasons for this type of pain and swelling in the joint. It is important to remember that different types of arthiritis occur at different ages and each one of them has a different outcome. Do not therefore worry unnecessarily if your doctor says that you have arthiritis.

## Types of knee injury?

Injury to the knee joint is quite common. As mentioned earlier, this is because the design of the knee makes it relatively unstable. It is also prone to injuries because of the stress the knee is subjected to. Causes and symptoms of common knee injuries have been listed before. Described below are the management options for these injuries.

- **Knee Sprain.** Minor twisting or bending of the knee result in a sprain which indicates that some tissues around the knee are pulled. Since pain due to sprain subsides within a few days to a week, you should consult a doctor immediately if the pain persists for more than three weeks, or if the swelling around the knee increases steadily. Your doctor may recommend rest in a plaster cast or crepe bandage for a few weeks.
- **Injury to semilunar cartilages.** The inner half-moon shaped or semilunar cartilage is more likely to be injured than the outer cartilage. Although cartilage injuries may seem insignificant, they can cause considerable damage to the structures inside the knee. Your doctor may suspect a cartilage tear if the pain does not subside in a few days. If the knee gets 'locked' in one position consult a doctor immediately to free it by manual manipulation.

Most injuries to the knee can cause repeated complaints. It is often difficult to pinpoint the exact nature of the damage by knowing the history of the injury and examination of the knee joint. Your doctor may then suggest a procedure called "arthroscopy" in which the doctor looks directly into the joint through a thin pencil like tube called the arthroscope. The arthroscope is introduced into the knee through a small cut in the skin. A video-camera is attached to the arthroscope, which shows the inside of the knee on a television. Through this procedure, your doctor will be able to view all the corners of the joint and may therefore be able to identify the cause of symptoms and nature of damage. In most cases, the fault within the joint can be corrected by "key-hole-surgery" with the help of small instruments inserted through a few more small cuts. This often avoids a major operation, enables quick recovery and reduces hospital stay to less than forty eight hours. Arthroscopy not only helps in diagnosing a problem that was not diagnosed earlier but also provides a method of performing surgery with minimum cutting. This technique is therefore a boon for patients with joint problems. However, presently arthroscopy facility is available only at few centres in India.

- **Injury to ligaments of the knee.** Minor ligament teat such as sprain may heal on its own. If the tear in the ligament is complete or more than one ligament is torn at a time, the knee may not regain its normal strength. You may feel unstable from the day of the injury itself. If the front middle ligament alone is torn, there may not be any symptoms soon after the injury. After a period of time, you may feel 'weak' on the injured side and knee pain may develop. Most people with torn ligaments feel better with regular special exercises and careful movements of the knee in day to day activities. However, if the weakness persists, your doctor may recommend a major operation to replace the torn ligament with a new ligament constructed from other body tissues.
- **Fractures and dislocations.** X-rays of the knee are necessary to diagnose the extent of bone(s) damage

due to the fracture. In most cases a major operation is necessary to fix the fractured pieces to their normal position with screws and steel plates. These steel plates result in normal movement at the knee. The pain and swelling subsides over a period of time.

- **Overuse injuries.** Knee injuries due to new or excessive physical activity is usually because of a mild problem in the 'design' of the knee. This problem may not routinely cause pain but can do so under stressful situations. It may not be necessary to give up physical activity that has resulted in knee pain. Instead, you should undertake strenuous physical activities only after receiving appropriate training and avoid excessive physical stress.

## How is Arthritis of the knee Treated?

Most often osteoarthritis of the knee is treated with analgesics (pain-reducing medicines), such as aspirin or acetaminophen, NSAlds such as ibuprofen; and exercises to restore joint movement and strengthen the knee. Losing excess weight can also help people with osteoarthritis. Rheumatoid arthritis of the knee may require a treatment plan that includes physical therapy and use of more powerful medications. In people with arthritis of the knee, a seriously damaged joint may need to be surgically replaced with an artificial one.

4

# PAIN (ARTHRITIS) OF THE SHOULDER

The shoulder joint is composed of three bones: the clavicle (collarbone), the scapula (shoulder blade), and the humerus (upper arm bone). Two joints facilitate shoulder movement. The acromioclavicular (AC) joint is located between the acromion (part of the scapula that forms the highest point of the shoulder) and the clavicle. The glenohumeral joint, commonly called the shoulder joint, is a ball-and-socket type joint that helps move the shoulder forward and backward and allows the arm to rotate in a circular fashion or hinge out and up away from the body. (The ball is the top, rounded portion of the upper arm bone or humerus; the socket. or glenoid, is a dish-shaped part of the outer edge of the scapula into which the ball fits.) The capsule is a soft tissue envelope that encircles the glenohumeral joint. It is lined by a thin, smooth synovial membrane.

The bones of the shoulder are held in place by muscles, tendons, and ligaments. Tendons are tough cords of tissue that attach the shoulder muscles to bone and assist the muscles in moving the shoulder. Ligaments attach shoulder bones to each other, providing stability. For example, the front of the joint capsule is anchored by three glenohumeral ligaments.

The rotator cuff is a structure composed of tendons that with associated muscles, holds the ball at the top of the humerus in the glenoid socket and provides mobility and strength to the shoulder joint. Two sac-like structures called bursae permit smooth gliding between bone, muscle and tendon. They cushion and protect the rotator cuff from the bony arch of the acromion. What are the Origin and Causes of Shoulder Problems?

The shoulder is the most movable joint in the body. However, it is an unstable joint because of the range of motion allowed. It is easily subject to injury because the ball of the upper arm is larger than the shoulder socket that holds it. To remain stable, the shoulder must be anchored by its muscles, tendons and ligaments. Some shoulder problems arise from the disruption of these soft tissues as a result of injury or from: overuse or underuse of the shoulder. Other problems arise from a degenerative process in which tissues break down and no longer function well.

Shoulder pain may be localized or may be referred to areas around the shoulder or down the arm. Disease within the body (such as gallbladder, liver, or heart disease, or disease of the cervical spine of the neck) also may generate pain that travels along nerves to the shoulder.

## What is Arthritis of the Shoulder?

Arthritis is a degenerative disease caused by either wear and tear (osteoarthritis) or an inflammation (rheumatoid arthritis) of one or more joints. Arthritis not only affects joints; it may secondarily affect supporting structures such as muscles, tendons and ligaments. What are the Signs of Shoulder Arthritis and how is it Diagnosed?

The usual signs of arthritis of the shoulder are pain, particularly over the AC joint, and a decrease in shoulder motion. A doctor may suspect the patient has arthritis when there is both pain and swelling in the joint. The diagnosis may be confirmed by a physical examination and x rays. Blood tests may be helpful for diagnosing rheumatoid arthritis, but other tests may be needed as well. Analysis of synovial fluid from the shoulder joint may be helpful in diagnosing some kinds of arthritis. Although arthroscopy permits direct visualization of damage to cartilage, tendons and ligaments, and may confirm a diagnosis, it is usually only done if a repair procedure is to be performed.

## How is Pain (Arthritis ) of the Shoulder Treated?

Most often osteoarthritis of the shoulder is treated with nonsteroidal anti- inflammatory drugs Such as aspirin or ibuprofen. (Rheumatoid arthritis of the shoulder may require physical therapy and additional medicine, such as corticosteroids.) When conservative treatment of osteoarthritis of the shoulder fails to relieve pain or improve function, or when there is severe deterioration of the joint causing parts to loosen and move out of place, shoulder joint replacement (arthroplasty) may provide better results. In this operation, a surgeon replaces the shoulder joint with an artificial ball for the humerus and a cap (glenoid) for the scapula. Passive shoulder exercises (where someone else moves the arm to rotate the shoulder joint) are started soon after surgery. Patients begin exercising on their own about 3 to 6 weeks after surgery. Eventually, stretching and strengthening exercises become a major part of the rehabilitation program. The success of the operation often depends on the condition of rotator cuff muscles prior to surgery and the degree to which the patient follows the exercise program.

5

# Rheumatoid Arthritis

Rheumatoid arthritis is a disease in which the body develops 'allergy' to some components of the blood. These components accumulate in the joints and some other parts of the body. The body's natural defence mechanism reacts adversely to this accumulation. The result is swelling and pain. Rheumatoid arthritis can cripple a person rapidly, is often extensive and may sometimes even be life-threatening. It is more common in women twenty to forty years of age and may run in families.

## Symptoms

Early symptoms of rheumatoid arthritis are fever with vague aches and pains in the body including the joints. After about four to six weeks the symptoms are more severe and the pain is present in several joints, especially the joints of the hands and feet. Knee is a major joint and is therefore usually affected. Walking may become difficult. If you do not walk enough, your thigh muscles may become wasted or thin. Rheumatoid arthritis may affect various systems of the body such as the eyes, lungs and the heart. Severity of the symptoms of rheumatoid arthritis is not constant. The symptoms may completely disappear and appear again after some time.

You should consult with a doctor as soon as possible if you have pain and swelling one or more joints. It is important to remember that all joint pains and swelling are not due to rheumatoid arthritis. What is the difference between osteoarthritis and rheumatoid arthritis?

Osteoarthritis usually begins after the age of forty years over a period of several years. It usually begins on joints on one side of the body. It usually affects joints in the knee, hips, hands, feet and the backbone. There are no associated symptoms such as fatigue, fever or loss of weight.

Rheumatoid arthritis starts between twenty five to forty years of age and the symptoms may appear and disappear without any warning. It affects joints on both sides of the body at the same time. It affects most joints including knuckles, wrist and elbows. Rheumatoid arthritis is usually accompanied with fever, weight loss and fatigue.

## Laboratory tests

Your doctor may recommend a test called teh R.A. factor. Although this test often helps in diagnosis, it is not always reliable. This is because it is occasionally positive in people who do not have rheumatoid arthritis. Your doctor will therefore diagnose your condition on the basis of history physical examination and laboratory tests.

## Management

The basic principles for management of rheumatoid arthritis and other associated diseases. These include:

- **Correct diagnosis.** Since rheumatoid arthritis is just one type of arthritis which involves multiple joints, it is important for you to consult with a doctor, especially a joint-disease specialist (Rheumatologist) and trust his/her judgment. Your doctor may not be able to make the diagnosis before six weeks.
- **Patient education.** Since rheumatoid arthritis is potentially crippling, it is important for you to

avoid anxiety. Your doctor will give you details about the course of the disease such as its fluctuating course, long-term treatment options, need to use more than one medicines which may have several adverse impacts, cost of treatment and the need to consult the doctor regularly. You can limit the adverse impacts of the disease by following your doctors recommendations.

- **Avoid treatment from doctors who are not qualified-** Several selfstyled doctors may promise your magic cure for rheumatoid arthritis. It is however important to remember that although some medicines may be partially effective for other types of arthritis, rheumatoid arthritis requires a well-planned management schedule.
- **Avoid steroids-** Steroids are chemical substances produced by some glands in the body. They are also available as medicines. Although steroids may give immediate relief you will require larger and larger dose to relieve symptoms over a period of time. They have serious side-effects on almost all parts of the body. Of these, weight-gain, swelling of the face, excess hair growth on the face, reduced vision due to cataract, ulcers and weakness of bones are more common.
- **Diet**-Rheumatoid arthritis does not require any special diet. Avoiding some food items are not likely to cure the disease. You may however have loss of appetite and anaemia. You should therefore eat a balanced diet preferably as small and frequent meals.
- **Moderate activity-**Bed rest is not necessary, except in early painful stages of the disease. Once this phase is over, you should start normal joint movements.
- **Physiotherapy-**It is very important to start

physiotherapy after the disease is controlled a little by medicines. Physiotherapy helps to regain joint mobility and strength. You can do the recommended exercise and heat therapy yourself after learning the correct technique from a qualified person.

## Principles of management

Correct diagnosis, preferably by a rheumatologist.
Education regarding the course of illness and adverse effects of the disease and its management options.
Acceptance that the disease is not curable.
Avoid steroids.
Eat small frequent balanced meals.
Do simple exercise after the painful stage subsides and gradually increase its duration.
Learn the correct technique of physiotherapy including exercise from a trained professional.
Avoid exercise from which you cannot recover within one hour.
Normal sexual activity can be practiced, especially when the painful stage subsides.
Avoid pregnancy during active phase of the disease.
Consult your doctor regularly for modifications in your treatment schedule depending upon you condition.
Surgery such as knee replacement if all other methods for joint mobility have failed.

## Exercise

Exercise help to relieve and prevent joint stiffness, muscle weakness, joint deformity and dependence on others. You should however avoid excessive bending of the joints. Increase the intensity and duration of the exercise gradually as you may feel tired after doing exercises to regain joint mobility and muscle strength. A simple rule is that you should recover from the 'strain' within one hour of exercises. It is important to find a correct balance between rest and exercise.

Three types of exercises help:

- those which maintain or increase joint mobility;
- those which improve muscle strength; and
- those which increase the general health and are beneficial to the heart and the lungs.
- **Marriage, sexual activity and motherhood-** Rheumatoid arthritis is a chronic disease which limits your ability to do normal work over a period of years. You can be sexual active although it may be difficult when you have joint pains. Although pregnancy is not contra-indicated in rheumatoid arthritis it is better to avoid pregnancy during the active phase of the disease when you require long-term medicines. Rarely the hip joint may be affected and therefore sexual activity and delivery may be difficult.
- **Regulate treatment schedule under doctor's guidance-**There is no common treatment for rheumatoid arthritis. Your doctor is likely to recommend a combination of medicines depending upon the severity of your disease, your body's acceptance of the medicines and their side-effects. Your doctor may have to modify the treatment schedule frequently in the initial stages till the correct combination and dose is achieved.
- **Surgery**-Your doctor may recommend surgery after other methods of preserving the joint and making it usable have falied. Knee joint replacement has become a very standred operation as it makes you mobile even after a prolonged illness.

## Moderate Treatment

When we use the term moderate it implies that it is a scaled down version of a radical treatment so far discussed.

Morning keep the bowel clean with the help of a non violent enema.

Herbal paste/juice can be combined with the vegetable juice of banana stem and/or ash pumkin.

If time permits spinal bath combined with hot foot bath may be taken for 15-20 minutes. Full bath in bearable cold water is to be followed.

With the above oral medicine the patient may proceed to his/her place of work/studies or continue with his/her light household chores.

10-11 a.m. Depending upon the convenience in the place of work/studies the patient may take some tender coconut water or some fresh non citrus fruits or some vegetable juice. If none of the above are available plain cold water is sufficient.

**Lunch at home :** some fresh vegetables and some conservatively cooked vegetables, with the usual garnishings of coconut scrapings, coriander leaves etc. may be taken. Better to avoid cereals.

If going to work some fruits or fresh vegetables are prescribed. Cooked food would have become very stale. Further he/she is expected to continue the work, also in the afternoon.

If at home a spinal bath with hot water foot bath may be taken in the afternoon. Those who go out for work/studies are advised to take a spinal bath with/without hot water foot bath without fail on return. Whatever help is needed for getting into the tub and getting up should be obtained. A glass of tender coconut water is an ideal drink in the evening.

Night dinner may consist of some unrefined cereals

and conservatevely cooked vegetables.

Before retiring to bed he/she may apply some edible herbal oil on the affected joints. This will be followed with an alternate hot and cold fomentation and at the end of it apply a stimulating wet pack on the affected joint(s).

6

# JUVENILE RHEUMATOID ARTHRITIS

Juvenile rheumatoid arthritis (JRA) is a different form of arthritis that causes joint inflammation and stiffness for more than 6 weeks in a child of 16 years of age or less. Inflammation causes redness, swelling, warmth, and soreness in the joints, although many children with JRA do not complain of joint pain. Any joint can be affected and inflammation may limit the mobility of affected joints. Doctors classify three kinds of JRA by the number of joints involved, the symptoms, and the presence or absence of certain antibodies in the blood. (Antibodies are special proteins made by the immune system.) These classifications help the doctor determine how the disease will progress.

**Pauciarticular:** (paw-see-are-tick-you-Iar): Pauciarti-cular means that four or fewer joints are affected. Pauciarticular is the most common form of JRA; about half of all children with JRA have this type. Pauciarticular disease typically affects large joints, such as the knees. Girls under the age of are most likely to develop this type of JRA.

Some children have special proteins in the blood called antinuclear antibodies (ANAs). Eye disease affects about 20 to 30 percent of children with pauciarticular JRA. Up to 80 percent of those with eye disease also test positive for ANA and the disease tends to develop at a particularly early age in these children. Regular examinations by an ophthalmologist (a doctor who specializes in eye diseases) are necessary to prevent serious eye problems such as iritis (inflammation of the iris) or uveitis (inflammation of the inner eye or uvea). Many children with pauciarticular disease outgrow arthritis by adulthood, although eye problems can continue and joint symptoms may recur in some people.

**Polyarticular:** About 30 percent of all children with JRA have polyarticular disease. In polyarticular disease, five or more joints are affected. The small joints, such as those in the hands and feet, are most commonly involved, but the disease may also affect large joints. Polyarticular JRA often is symmetrical, that is, it affects the same joint on both sides of the body. Some children with polyarticular disease have a special kind of antibody in their blood called IgM rheumatoid factor (RF). These children often have a more severe form of the disease, which doctors consider to be the same as adult rheumatoid arthritis.

**Systemic:** Besides joint swelling, the systemic form of JRA is characterized by fever and a light pink rash, and may also affect internal organs such as the heart, liver, spleen and lymph nodes. Doctors sometimes call it Still's disease. Almost all children with this type of JRA test negative for both RF and ANA. The systemic form affects 20 percent of all children with JRA. A small percentage of these children develop arthritis in many joints and can have severe arthritis that continues into adulthood.

JRA is an autoimmune disorder, which means that the body mistakenly identifies some of its own cells and tissues as foreign. The immune system, which normally helps to fight off harmful, foreign substances such as bacteria or viruses, begins to attack healthy cells and tissues. The result is inflammation-marked by redness, heat, pain and swelling. Doctors do not know why the immune system goes awary in children who develop JRA. Scientists suspect that it is a two-step process. First something in a child's genetic makeup gives them a tendency to develop JRA; and then an environmental factor, such as a virus, triggers the development of JRA.

The most common symptom of all types of JRA is persistent joint swelling, pain, and stiffness that typically is worse in the morning or after a nap. The pain may limit movement of the affected joint although many children, especially younger ones, will not complain of pain. JRA commonly affects the knees and joints in the hands and feet. One of the earliest signs of JRA may be limping in the morning because of an affected knee. Besides joint symptoms, children with systemic JRA have a high fever and a light pink rash. The rash and fever may appear and disappear very quickly. Systemic JRA also may cause the lymph nodes located in the neck and other parts of the body to swell. In some cases (less than half), internal organs including the heart and very rarely, the lungs may be involved. Eye inflammation is a potentially severe complication that sometimes occurs in children with pauciarticular IRA. Eye diseases such as iritis and uveitis often are not present until some time after a child first develops JRA. Typically, there are periods when the symptoms of JRA are better or disappear (remissions) and times when symptoms are worse (flares). JRA is different in each child-some may have just one or two flares and never have symptoms again, while others experience many flares or even have symptoms that never go away.

**The Difference between JRA and Adult RA:** The main difference between juvenile and adult rheumatoid arthritis is that many people with JRA outgrow the illness, while adults usually have lifelong symptoms. Studies estimate that by adulthood, JRA symptoms disappear in more than half of all affected children. Additionally, unlike rheumatoid arthritis in an adult, JRA may affect bone development as well as the child's growth. Another difference between JRA and adult rheumatoid arthritis is the percentage of people who are positive for RF. About 70 to 80 percent of all adults with rheumatoid arthritis are positive for RF, but fewer than half of all children with rheumatoid arthritis are RF positive. Presence of RF indicates an increased chance that 1RA will continue into adulthood.

7

# Exercise for Arthritics/Pain

Many arthritics shirk from exercise because they think it would be terribly painful in their condition. But in arthritis. if moving hurts, not moving destroys. Incorrect moving harms but intelligent moving heals. Use it or lose it!

Exercise helps keep you fit and slim. If you have arthritis, it helps keep your joints, muscles and bones healthy. Exercise also gives you more energy to keep up with daily activities. However, the pain and swelling of arthritis may complicate your workout routine, and hence the need for a trained physical therapist. A yoga teacher can train you in movements with proper joint alignment which help bring deformed joints back to normal position as appropriate muscles are lengthened and strengthened.

The amount and form of exercise recommended for each individual will vary depending on which joints are involved, the amount of inflammation, how stable the joints are, and whether a joint replacement procedure has been done. A skilled physician who is knowledgeable about the medical and rehabilitation needs of people with arthritis, working with a physical therapist also familiar with the needs of people with arthritis, can design an exercise plan for each patient.

## Should People With Arthritis Exercise?

Yes. Studies have shown that exercise helps people

with arthritis in many ways. Exercise reduces joint pain and stiffness and increases flexibility, muscle strength, and endurance. It also helps with weight reduction and contributes to an improved sense of well-being.

## How does Exercise Fit into a Treatment Plan for People with Arthritis?

Exercise is one part of a comprehensive arthritis treatment plan. Treatment plans also may include rest and relaxation, proper diet, medication, and instruction about proper use of joints and ways to conserve energy (that is, not waste motion) as well as the use of pain relief methods.

## How does a Person with Arthritis Start an Exercise Program?

People with arthritis should discuss exercise options with their doctors. Most doctors recommend exercise for their patients. Many people with arthritis begin with easy, range-of-motion exercises and low-impact aerobics. People with arthritis can participate in a variety of, but not all, sports and exercise programs. The doctor will know which, if any, sports are off limits.

The doctor may have suggestions about how to get started or may refer the patient to a physical therapist. It is best to find a physical therapist who has experience working with people who have arthritis. The therapist will design an appropriate home exercise program and teach clients about pain-relief methods, proper body mechanics (placement of the body for a given task, such as lifting a heavy box), joint protection, and conserving energy.

### What Types of Exercise are most Suitabsle for Someone with Arthritis?

- Isometric Exercises consist of tightening your muscles without moving your joints. Example: From an upright sitting or standing position, press the palms of both hands together with all your might, as if you were trying to press communion wafers. This strengthens your arm muscles.
- Isotonic Exercises strengthen muscles by using a light weight or other resistance. Several studies now show that if you improve muscle strength, you decrease pain. An example of isotonic exercises for your thighs: Sit in a chair high enough that you can swing your leg. Keep your thigh on the chair and straighten out your knee. Hold a few seconds. Then bend your knee back as far as possible. Repeat with the other knee.
- Range of Motion Exercises reduce stiffness and help keep your joints flexible by making sure they are regularly moved the full extent of their range. Example for your thumbs: Open your hand with your fingers straight. Reach your thumb across your palm until it touches the base of the little finger. Then stretch your thumb out and repeat. Keep in mind that normal every day activities, such as cleaning, climbing stairs, dressing, bathing, cooking, lifting, or bending do not move your joints through their entire range of motion. If your joints are very painful and swollen, do not forgo your exercises. Simply move them gently through their range of motion.
- Aerobic exercises improve cardiovascular fitness, help control weight, and improve overall function. Weight control can be important to people who have arthritis because extra weight puts extra

pressure on many joints. Some studies show that aerobic exercise can reduce inflammation in some joints.

## How to Get Started

- Discuss exercise plans with your doctor.
- Start with supervision from a physical therapist.
- Apply heat to sore joints (optional; many people with arthritis start their exercise program this way).
- Stretch and warm up with range-of-motion exercises.
- Start strengthening exercises slowly with small weights (a kilo weight can make a big difference).
- Progress slowly.
- Use cold packs after exercising (optional; many people with arthritis complete their exercise routine this way).
- Add aerobic exercise.
- Consider appropriate recreational exercise (after doing range of-motion. strengthening, and aerobic exercise). Fewer injuries to arthritic joints occur during recreational exercise if it is preceded by strengthening and aerobic exercise that gets your body in the best condition possible.
- Ease off if joints become painful. inflamed, or red and work with your doctor to find the cause and eliminate it.
- Choose the exercise program you enjoy most and make it a habit.
- Avoid weight bearing activities such as climbing stairs and prolonged walking

## Pain Relief Methods?

There are known methods to stop pain for short

periods of time. This temporary relief can make it easier for people who have arthritis to exercise. The following methods have worked for many people:

- ☞ Moist heat supplied by warm towels, hot packs, a bath, or a shower can be used at home for 15 to 20 minutes three times a day to relieve symptoms. A health professional can use short waves, microwaves, and ultrasound to deliver deep heat to noninflamed joint areas. Deep heat is not recommended for patients with acutely inflamed joints. Deep heat is often used around the shoulder to relax tight tendons prior to stretching exercises.
- ☞ Cold supplied by a bag of ice or frozen vegetables wrapped in a towel helps to stop pain and reduce swelling when used.
- ☞ For 10 to 15 minutes at a time, it is often used for acutely inflamed joints. People who have Raynauds phenomenon should not use this method.
- ☞ Application of a muscle ointment at night before going to bed helps people with arthritis to feel much better all day. They aren't stiff when they wake up in the morning
- ☞ Massages, on account of the gentle warmth they produce, alleviate the pain considerably. In case of stiff joints, massage with a mixture of warm coconut and mustard oil and camphor.

Work the muscles that are attached to the tendons leading to your painful joints. For example if you have arthritis in your hands then work the forearms from the wrists to the elbows, using a compression technique. To do this use withe the heel of your hand, your thumb or your elbow to press down on the muscle and hold it for several seconds, then release. For arthritis of the foot, work the calf and the front to the leg.

- ☞ Mobilisation therapies include traction (gentle,

steady pulling), massage, and manipulation (using the hands to restore normal movement to stiff joints). When done by a trained professional, these methods can help control pain and increase joint motion and muscle and tendon flexibility.

☞ TENS (transcutaneous electrical nerve stimulation) and biofeedback are two additional methods that may provide some pain relief, but many patients find that they cost too much money and take too much time.

☞ Relaxation therapy also helps reduce pain. Patients can learn to release the tension in their muscles to relieve pain. Physical therapists may be able to teach relaxation techniques.

☞ Acupuncture is a traditional Chinese method of pain relief. A medically qualified acupuncturist places needles in certain sites. Researchers believe that the needles stimulate deep sensory nerves that tell the brain to release natural painkillers (endorphins). Acupressure is similar to acupuncture, but pressure is applied to the acupuncture sites instead of using needles.

## How Often Should People with Arthritis Exercise?

☞ Range-of-motion exercises can be done daily and should be done at least every other day.

☞ Strengthening exercises also can be done daily and should be done at least every other day unless you have severe pain or swelling in your joints.

☞ Endurance exercises should be done for 20 to 30 minutes three times a week unless you have severe pain or swelling in your joints.

## What Type of Strengthening Program is Best?

This varies depending on personal preference, the type of arthritis involved, and how active the inflammation is. Strengthening one's muscles can help take the burden off painful joints. Strength training can be done with small weights, exercise machines, isometrics, elastic bands, and resistive water exercises: Correct positioning is critical, because if done incorrectly, strengthening exercises can cause muscle tears, more pain, and more joint swelling.

## Are There Different Exercises for People with Different Types of Arthritis?

There are many types of arthritis. Experienced doctors, physical therapists and occupational therapists can recommend exercises that are particularly helpful for a specific type of arthritis. Doctors and therapists also know specific exercises for particularly painful joints. There may be exercises that are offlimits for people with a particular type of arthritis or when joints are swollen and inflamed. People with arthritis should discuss their exercise plans with a doctor. Doctors who treat people with arthritis include rheumatologists, general practitioners, family doctors, internists, and rehabilitation specialists.

## How Much Exercise is too Much?

Most experts agree that if exercise causes pain that lasts for more than 1 hour, it is too much. People with arthritis should work with their physical therapist or doctor to adjust their exercise program when they notice any of the following signs of too much exercise:

- ☞ Unusual or persistent fatigue
- ☞ Increased weakness
- ☞ Decreased range of motion

- ☞ Increased joint swelling
- ☞ Continuing pain (pain that lasts more than 1 hour after exercising)

## Exercises to Keep Your Muscles from Becoming Stiff

If you have trouble sitting for long periods of time, try the following exercises devised by physiologist Mary Sampey. These are useful for keeping your muscles from becoming stiff. Always begin these exercises by sitting comfortably, but alertly in your chair, feet flat on the floor and hands resting on your thighs. Each exercise should be done as tolerated, however only a few minutes at a time are necessary to make a difference.

Neck Stretch: Gently bend your head forward, then to each side. Repeat 2 to 3 times.

Arm Reaches: Sitting up straight, stretch your arms over your head. Reach first with your right arm, then with your left, as if you were climbing a ladder. If you can repeat this set of stretches 9 to 10 times.

Wrist Rolls. Gently rotate your right wrist. Circle in one direction several times, then reverse the rotation. Repeat with your left wrist.

Shoulder Rolls: Sitting up straight, slowly roll your shoulders in a circle. Roll forward 2 to 3 times, then backward.

Side Circles: Stretch arms out to your sides. Circle forward 10 times, starting with small, tight circles that gradually become broader and looser. Repeat with reverse circling.

Lower Back Stretch: Slowly bend your upper body toward your knees as low as comfortably possible, letting your arms rest on your lower legs or around your ankles. Return to the sitting position, then repeat 1 to 2 times.

Upper Body Stretch: Visualize a wire attached to the top of your head, gently stretching your body upward.

Hold the stretch for a few moments, then relax. Repeat 2 to 3 times.

Tiptoe Stretches: Sit with your feet flat on the floor. Leaving the front part of the foot (ball and toes) on the floor, slowly raise the heel of your right foot into a comfortable stretch. You should feel a slight stretch in your calf as well. Then lower your heel back to the floor. Repeat 2 to 3 times with your right foot.

Heel Stretches: Sit with feet flat on the floor. Leaving the heel of your foot on the floor, slowly raise the front part of your foot a few inches until you feel gently stretch in your ankle and calf. Then lower the front part of your foot back to the floor. Repeat 2 to 3 times, then switch to the left foot.

8

# Diet and Nutritional Supplements

If you thought that all you could do to combat arthritis was to pop painkillers and suffer, you obviously have not been talking to the right people. There are enough good studies to show that diet therapy may improve symptoms in some cases.

- Corn, wheat, cow's milk, pork, oranges, oats, eggs, beef, coffee, cheese, grapefruit, lemon,. tomato, groundnuts and soya are the foods most likely to cause arthritis. Makes sense to avoid them, doesn't it?

  (Note: Animal products such as meat and cows' dairy products contain a fatty acid called Arachidonic acid that greatly contributes to the inflammation of joints)
- Diet should be planned on alkaline lines so as to rid the system of its toxicity. A diet predominated by raw salad, sprouts and cooked vegetables is effective in this regard. At least one meal a day should be exclusively comprised of raw salad, sprouts and fruits. Excess salt should be avoided as salt will cause more water to be retained in the body and joint pains will increase.
- A weekly fast for a day or two, or at least a juice fast for a couple of days, is extremely beneficial. Constipation should be avoided since any increase in toxicity only irritates the joints and causes further inflammation.

- Make it a point to include cabbage, carrot, cucumber, lettuce, onion, radish, beet root, cauliflower, banana, and green leafy vegetables in your salad or in your vegetable menu. Eat enough garlic as it is very effective in removing toxins and stimulating blood circulation. Above all, avoid all refined foods, flesh foods, eggs, milk and milk products and fried and spicy foods.
- Tomatoes, white potatoes, eggplant and green bell peppers are members of the Night Shade Vegetable Family. These vegetables contain a chemical called Soltanine that may aggravate arthritis sufferers. Elimination of these vegetables for one week and the reintroduction of one - of these at a time, may determine any possible allergic reaction.
- Omega-3 polyunsaturated fatty acids (PUFAs) could help prevent and treat a wide range of diseases, including arthritis. The daily requirement is probably around a teaspoon of essential fatty acids a day. Fish is a rich source of omega-3 PUF and also of eicosapentaenoic acid (EPA). EPA greatly reduces inflammation and contributing allergic responses. If you are a vegetarian, use Flax Seed Oil (Omega 3 oi1) or canola oil (high in a plant form of omega-3 alpha linoleic fatty acid).
- Take in plenty of berries: (cherries, blueberries). These are rich in flavonoids that inhibit histaminic release and reduces the inflammatory response.
- Take enough of vitamin C daily. This vitamin assists in decreasing histaminic levels and inflammation while providing anti-oxidant effects. Vitamin C is a marker for fruits and vegetables rich in other healing compounds. Therefore, stick with foods high in vitamin C rather than supplements. Indian gooseberry (aamla) is one of the best known sources of vitamin C.

- ☞ Enzymes: Especially Trypsin, Bromelain and Quercetin along with Vitamin C and Flavanoids, have been found to provide a wider use for individuals with Rheumatoid Arthritis than non-steroidal drugs such as aspirin.
- ☞ Acidophillus: Provides friendly bacteria to balance abnormal intestinal flora common with Rheumatoid Arthritis sufferers.
- ☞ Because RA follows a pattern of flare ups, it's natural to suspect you are allergic to what you have just eaten. Keep a daily chart of your diet and your reactions; this will help you eliminate the food type to which you are allergic.

## Fat Intake & Arthritis

According to Prevention, the immune substances that inflame your joints are made from the kind of fat you eat. Linoleic acid - the predominant polyunsaturated fat in most vegetable oils such as soybean. corn oil, safflower and sunflower, generate some of the most inflammatory immune substances. Therefore change your fatty-acid profile to a less inflammatory one. Canola oil is once again preferable. It will also help keep your cholesterol profile in check.

A low-fat diet (keep fat at 20 percent of total calories) has been found to decrease morning stiffness by 50 percent and improve walking time by 30 percent.

## Suggested Calcium & Vitamin D Intake

On the basis of the most current information available, optimal calcium intake is estimated to be 400 mg/day (birth to 6 months) to 600 mg/day (6 to 12 months) in infants; 800 mg/day in young children (1 to 5 years) and 800 to 1,200 mg/day for older children (6 to 10 years); 1,200 to

1,500 mg/day for adolescents and young adults (11 to 24 years); 1,000 mg/day for women between 25 and 50 years; 1,200 to 1,500 mg/day for pregnant or lactating women; and 1,000 mg/day for postmenopausal women on estrogen replacement therapy and 1,500 mg/day for postmenopausal women not on estrogen therapy. Recommended daily intake for men is 1,000 mg/day (25 to 65 years). For all women and men over 65, daily intake is recommended to be 1,500 mg/day, although further research is needed in this age group. These guidelines are based upon calcium from the diet plus any calcium taken in supplemental form.

Also remember that adequate vitamin D is essential for optimal calcium absorption. More so in osteoarthritis which breaks down cartilage in a joint, causing the underlying bone to be subjected to greater stress. Low levels of vitamin D may impair the ability of bone to respond to this increased wear and tear. Take multivitamin with at least 4000 IU of vitamin D.

- ☞ Phosphorus is an element which takes out excess of calcium from body. So, make sure its proper bone should be consumed.
- ☞ If there is RA or any related disorder, diet should be suggested by a qualified nutritional therapist.

# 9

# WHAT IS OSTEOARTHRITIS?

Osteoarthritis is destruction of the smooth cartilage covering the ends of the bones. This destruction is similar to the wear and tear of moving machines. It usually starts in the middle age without any specific cause. You may have seen elderly persons walking like a duck, or using a stick to walk. Most of these people suffer from osteoarthritis.

## Stages

In early stages there is pain or catch in the knee while:

- getting up from siting position or
- changing position of the knee after a period of rest in one position.

  In later stages, pain is almost constant and becomes worse on exertion. At this stage the pain is relieved by :

- rest;
- pain killer medicines; or
- oil massage.

In advanced stage, walking is difficult and often needs a lot of effort. Going up and down the stairs is especially very difficult. The knee may appear 'swollen' and thigh may appear thin. The shape of the legs changes and the knee bows outwards. At this stage, the gait changes and there may be sideways lurch at every step.

## Causes

Common causes of osteoarthritis are:

☞ Wear-and-tear due to prolonged use of the joint (This is the commonest cause of osteoarthritis);

☞ Defect in quality of the cartilage such as in a disease called pseudogout;

☞ Defect in alignment of the articulating surfaces;

☞ Loose structures inside the joint such as a loose cover of the meniscus;

☞ Old injury; and

☞ Previous infection.

## Risk groups

Osteoarthritis may run in families. It is more common in obese people and those who use the knee excessively such as for sports, standing for a long time or working for long hours with knee in extreme positions. Osteoarthritis is 10 time more common in females than in the males. People with bowed legs develop osteoarthritis much earlier.

## Symptoms

Osteoarthritis of the knee is more common among people above fifty years of age, especially the obese. Most people with osteoarthritis complain of pain and/or creaking sound in the knee.

Many people who believe that knee pain means beginning of old age do not always consult with a doctor. It is important to remember that knee pain can occur at all ages and some causes are curable. Also, there are some diseases which may start as a mild pain but rapidly progress to destroy the knee joint. Early diagnosis and timely management that can prevent the progress of an otherwise progressive disease.

## When to consult with a doctor?

You should consult with a doctor, especially orthopedic surgeon if you have:

- Pain or stiffness in one joint only or if one joint is affected more than the other;
- Repeated swelling of the knee with pain;
- Symptoms suggestive of a mechanical fault as sudden clicking, something either moving or loose inside the joint.
- Recent bowing of the legs with pain or the inner side of the knee.
- Walking about within the house is difficult due to pain.

## Management

Osteoarthritis is not curable. Once it starts, it remains for rest of the life. However, you can relieve the symptoms and minimise disability with timely treatment. Management of osteoarthritis is through

- non-surgical methods in early stages and
- surgical methods in advanced stages.

## Non-Surgical Management

The patient has to do the following for non-surgical management of osteoarth ritis.

**Patient education.** You may start worrying about being crippled because of arthritis. Your doctor will, therefore, give you a very true picture of your condition which will help lessen your fears and anxiety.

**Weight reduction.** Regular and adequate exercise may be a problem if you have difficulty in walking. You may, however, do cycling or swimming regularly. It is, therefore, important to modify your diet and avoid high calorie foods such as sugar, sweets, rice, potato, oil or ghee.

## Avoid the following which put excessive stress on the knee

- Sitting on the floor, in low chairs, sofa or beds.
- Squatting, sitting cross-legged and using Indian style toilets.
- Exercises in which you have stand or walk for a long time.

## You may get relief by

- Doing exercises where you can sit on a chair or stool.
- Doing specific exercises to build up the muscles around the knee for providing support to the 'weak' knee.
- Occasional use of medicines to relieve pain. Paracetamol is a safer medicine.

## Surgical Management

Three types of surgeries are recommended for management of osteoarthritis. These include:

- arthroscopy;
- correction of the alignment of the knee; and
- changing the knee joint. None of these surgeries cure osteoarthritis. Your doctor may recommend anyone of these options depending upon the condition of your knee.
- **Arthroscopy.** Your doctor may recommend if you either have
- mechanical problems such as something stuck or loose inside the joint or
- repeated swelling of the knee joint. Although the relief may be partial or temporary, it is often recommended because it is a safe and 'minor' procedure.

As mentioned earlier, your doctor can view the inside of the knee directly through an arthroscope and assess the condition of the cartilage covering the bone-ends and the semi-lunar cartilages. Your doctor will also be able to remove (a) any loose or torn pieces of semi-lunar or articular cartilages or

- ☞ loose or over-grown tissue lining the knee. The joint will then be washed thoroughly with saline water to completely remove damaged pieces.
- ☞ **Correction of alignment of the knee.** Your doctor may suggest a surgery called High Tibial Osteotomy (HTO) to correct the alignment of the knee. This surgery is usually recommended if you have painful osteoarthritis of the knee with bowing of the legs. When your legs are bowed, more body weight passes through the inner side than the outer side of the knee. During the surgery the bone just below the knee is cut and realigned so that the more body weight passes through the outer side of the knee. After this surgery more than seventy percent patients have relief from pain for almost eight to ten years. It is effective for mild to moderate arthritis, and people who are either young or not obese.

High tibial osteotomy or HTO is a major surgery and requires a plaster cast for a month after the operation. You can however start walking to the toilet with the plaster about one week after the surgery. Your doctor will also recommend physiotherapy for a few weeks after the cast is removed.

- ☞ **Changing the knee joint.** This is a relatively new technique in which the damaged ends of the bones of the knee joint are removed and replaced with artificial parts. A cup-like part is fixed on the end of the thigh bone and a plate-like part is fixed on the end of the leg bone with a special glue called bone-cement. The new parts of the knee are smooth and therefore there is not pain during normal movements of the joint. Although this surgery gives instant relief from pain, it is not always effective. You may have to observe several restrictions in movements so that the new joint may last for five to eight years. Also, the artificial knee joint is very expensive. This surgery is usually recommended for people who are not able to walk within the house also.

10

# Other Conditions Like Arthritis

These are some disorders which resemble to arthritis.

## Bursitis and Tendinitis

Bursitis and Tendinitis result from irritation caused by injuring or overusing a joint. Bursitis affects a small sac that helps muscles more easily. Tendinitis affects the tendons that attach muscle to bone.

## Polymyalgia Rheumatica (PMR)

This rheumatic disorder causes muscle pain, aching and stiffuess in the neck and shoulders, lower back, thighs and hips. It can last a few months or many years. Most people experience severe stiffuess in the morning.

## Fibromyalgia

People with fibromyalgia feel pain and stiffuess in muscles and tendons, especially in the neck and upper back. The pain can last for weeks, months or years. The symptoms may disappear by themselves. This condition often is related to sleep problems, poor conditioning, or an old injury. In fact, fibromyalgia is a chronic disorder characterized by widespread musculoskeletal pain, fatigue and tenderness in localized areas of the neck, spine, shoulders, and hips called "tender points." People with this syndrome may also experience sleep disturbances, morning stiffness, irritable bowel syndrome, anxiety and other symptoms. It primarily occurs in women of childbearing age, but children, the elderly and men may also be affected.

Although the cause of fibromyalgia is unknown, some scientists believe that an injury or trauma may cause the syndrome. This injury may affect the central nervous system. Fibromyalgia may be associated with changes in muscle metabolism, such as decreased blood flow, causing fatigue and decreased strength. Others believe an infectious agent, such as a virus in susceptible people, may trigger the syndrome, but no such agent has been identified.

Fibromyalgia is difficult to diagnose because many of the symptoms mimic those of other diseases. As per the criteria laid down a person is considered to have fibromyalgia if he or she has widespread pain for at least 3 months in combination with tenderness in at least 11 of 18 specific tender point sites.

Treatment of fibromyalgia requires a comprehensive approach. The physician, physiotherapist, and others in the medical support system, as well as the patient may all play an active role in the management of fibromyalgia. Studies have shown that aerobic exercise, such as swimming and walking, improves muscle fitness and reduces muscle pain and tenderness. Heat and massage may also give short-tern relief. Antidepressant medications may help elevate mood, improve quality of sleep and relax muscles. Fibromyalgia patients may benefit ftom a combination of exercise, medication, physical therapy and relaxation.

## Paget's Disease

This is a type of disorder in which the calcium in bones spreads unevenly. The bones most commonly affected are in the lower back, pelvis, tailbone, skull, and long bones of the legs. It is slightly more common in men than in women. It often begins between the ages of 50 and 70. Back pain may be a symptom, but most often there are no obvious symptoms. Paget's disease usually is discovered on a x-ray or bone scan done for reasons other than pain.

### Food Poisoning and Reiter's Syndrome

Food or water spoiled by salmonella or certain other bacteria can lead to a form of arthritis called Reiter's Syndrome. People who develop this rare kind of arthritis seem to have a defect in their body's defense system. This makes them more likely to develop arthritis in response to certain infections.

# 11

# ANKYLOSING SPONDYLITIS

This form of arthritis causes the joints in the spine to become stiff and swollen. In certain cases stiff joints can fuse (grow together). The most common symptoms are pain and stiffuess in the buttocks and lower back (particularly in the morning) that continue for more than three months. Ankylosing spondylitis is most common in men and often begins between the ages of 20 and 40.

So it is clear that ankylosing spondylitis primarily affects the spine or back. The joints and ligaments that normally permit the spine to move become inflamed and stiff. The bones of the spine may grow together, causing the spine to become rigid and inflexible. Other joints such as the hips, shoulders, knees, or ankles also may become involved. Heredity seems to playa role in determining who gets ankylosing spondylitis as it is noticed that approximately one in five people affected by ankylosing spondylitis have a relative with the same disorder. A gene called HLA-B27 is present in over 90 percent of people with ankylosing spondylitis. Ten to fifteen percent of individuals who inherit the gene will demonstrate ankylosing spondylitis.

Almost all people with ankylosing spondylitis can expect to lead normal and productive lives. Despite the chronic nature of the illness, only a few people with ankylosing spondylitis will become severely disabled. The management of pain and the control of inflammation can reduce the daily problems that may occur with ankylosing spondylltis. By watching posture and Almost always involved body position and by doing exercises daily, the individual can control many of the effects of the disease.

Symptoms of ankylosing spondylitis appear most frequently in young men between the ages of 16 and 35. It is less common in women, whose symptoms are often milder and more difficult to diagnose. About five percent of ankylosing spondylitis begins in childhood; boys are more likely to have it than girls.

When children develop ankylosing spondylitis, it usually begins in the hips, knees and bottoms of heels or big toes and may later progress to involve the spine. The inflammation in ankylosing spondylitis usually starts with the back pain. Typically, symptoms lessen with movement and exercise. Over a period of time, pain and stiffness may progress into the upper spine and even into the chest and neck. Ultimately, the inflammation can cause the sacroiliac and vertebral bones to whole spine become rigid. Similarly, the bones in the chest may fuse, causing a loss of normal chest expansion when breathing. The hips, shoulders, knees or ankles also may become inflamed and painful and eventually lose their mobility. The heels may become affected, making it uncomfortable to stand or walk on hard surfaces. Ankylosing spondylitis is a systemic disease, meaning it affects the entire body in some people. It can cause fever, loss of appetite and fatigue and it can damage other organs besides the joints, such as the lungs, heart and eyes.

The eye is the most common organ affected by ankylosing spondylitis. Eye inflammation (iritis) occurs from time to time in one fourth of people with ankylosing spondylitis. Iritis results in a red, painful eye that worsens by looking at bright light. It is a serious condition requiring immediate medical attention by an ophthalmologist. Less frequently, ankylosing spondylitis may be associated with a scaly skin condition called psoriasis. In rare cases, ankylosing spondylitis may cause problems with the heart, lungs, or intestines. Symptoms similar to that seen in ankylosing spondylitis also may occur along with such conditions as psoriasis, inflammatory bowel disease, or Reiter's syndrome. Doctors usually base their diagnosis of ankylosing spondylitis on symptoms (pain, stiffness) and x -rays showing involvement of the sacroiliac joint at the back of the pelvis. If the symptoms and x-rays suggest ankylosing spondylitis, but the diagnosis is uncertain, the doctor may perform a blood test to check you for the HLA - B27 gene. About 90 percent of people diagnosed with ankylosing spondylitis do test positive for this gene. Treatment for ankylosing spondylitis should be , designed to reduce pain and stiffness, prevent deformities and maintain the normal activities.

# 12

# Back Pain: Causes/ Symptoms/Investigations

Back, having so many parts, makes easy to develop a problem into itself. Anything that puts pressure on the back muscles or nerves can cause pain. Any illness or damage to the spine also can cause pain. The cause of most acute back pain is unknown, but probably is due to minor strains, sprains, and overuse. Emotional stress may add to the pain, especially since it slows the rate of recovery. Other possible causes of back pain include a ruptured intervertebral disc, spinal stenosis, osteoarthritis, anykylosing spondylitis, an injury or accident, rheumatic-related problems or other conditions.

Many of the problems that cause back pain are the result of injury and degeneration of the intervertebral disc. Degeneration is a process where wear and tear causes deterioration. The disc is subjected to different types of stress as we use our backs each day. Bending over results in compression of the disc and may also cause the disc to bulge backwards towards the spinal canal and nerves. The facet joints must also shift to allow the bending to occur. Twisting and bending together is perhaps the greatest stress on the parts of the spine, especially the disc.

Probably, the earliest of changes that occur in the disc are tears in the annulus portion of the intervertebral disc. The annulus is a large round ligament and the tears in the annulus heal the same way as the tears in other ligaments do, that is by scar formation. Scar tissue is not as strong as normal tissue. The repeated cycle of many annular tears healing by scar tissue leads to the disc that finally begins to degenerate.

## What happens when the disc begins to degenerate?

As the degeneration of the disc progresses the nucleus pulposus loses some of its water content. It becomes stiff and loses the ability to act as a shock absorber. The process may continue until the disc is collapsed. Bone spurs may form as the body's response to this degeneration. These spurs are thought to be the result of excess motion at the spinal segment. Eventually, bone spurs form around the nerves of the spine as well.

One of the most dramatic injuries to the lumbar spine is the Herniated Disc. In this injury, a tear in the annular ligament allows the nucleus pulposus to squeeze into the spinal canal. If the disc material compresses the nerve root, there is pain, numbness, and weakness in the areas supplied by the nerve. There is a considerable amount of evidence to suggest that it's not only the pressure that plays a part in the symptoms from a herniated disc. The nucleus material that is squeezed out against the nerve seems to set up an inflammatory response in the nerves causing pain.

## Symptoms

Low back pain can be divided into two main types:

- Mechanical Type pain
- Compressive Type pain

Mechanical type back pain results from inflammation caused by irritation or injury to the disc, the facet joints the ligaments or the muscles of the back. A common cause of mechanical pain is disc degeneration. A typical muscle strain, or lumbar strain, can also be the cause of mechanical type symptoms. Mechanical type back pain usually starts near the lower spine. Mechanical type pain may also spread to include the buttock and thigh areas. It rarely extends below the knee.

Compressive or neurogenic (meaning nerve related) type pain occurs when the nerve roots that leave the spine are irritated or pinched. A common cause of compressive pain is a herniated disc. The nerves that leave the lower lumbar spine join to form the sciatic nerve. This nerve provides sensation and controls the muscles of the lower leg. Pressure or irritations on the nerve roots of the lumbar spine that come together to form the sciatic nerve can interfere with the normal function of the sciatic nerve. One of the earliest signs of pressure on a nerve root is numbness in the area supplied by the nerve. Pain is commonly felt in the same area, usually extending below the knee to the foot. In cases where there is pressure on a nerve root as it comes out of the spine, it is not unusual for the back itself to be painless. This can be confusing at times since there is no back pain but the problem is located in the lumbar spine. Finally, the muscles that the nerve controls may become weak and the reflexes may disappear. This is because the pressure on the nerve roots interferes with the signals from the brain to the muscles. There is no signal going from the brain to the muscle to tell it to contract.

Spinal stenosis can also cause compressive type pain. In some people, degeneration of the spine can result in a narrowing of the spinal canal- the bony tube where the spinal nerves are located. This causes all of the nerves within the spinal canal to become inflamed, and fail to work properly. One problem that occurs when the tube is too small, is that the nerves can not get enough blood supply to work properly. The nerves may be normal when the body is at rest, but once it is active the nerves need more blood flow to get more oxygen. If the tube is too tight, the blood supply cannot increase. One of the symptoms of this cause is numbness. It may be in one or both the legs. The numbness may become worse with activities. The pain can involve both of the lower extremities. The pain becomes worse on walking and gets better after short periods of rest. Weakness of the muscles of both legs may also occur, and again, this may get worse when activity increases.

In very few cases, a disc herniation can be so big that it fills the entire spinal canal. The immediate pressure on the nerves in the spine may cause paralysis of the muscles that control the bowels and bladder. When the control over the bowels or bladder is lost, it is better to contact the physician immediately. **If the back pain is accompanied by any of the following, the doctor should be consulted:**

- weakness or numbness in one or both legs
- pain going down one leg below the knee
- back pain from a fall or injury
- back pain accompanied by fever without
- pain that continues to interrupt sleep after three nights
- back pain that remains after six weeks of home treatment

## Diagnosis

To enable the doctor to diagnose the problem correctly the complete history of the back pain should be provided. The doctor may ask a number of questions as listed below:

- What are the symptoms?
- What kinds of aches or pains?
- Where exactly is the pain?
- Where is the pain the most severe?
- When did the pain begin?
- How long it lasts?
- Did-something specific cause the back pain, such as an accident or injury?
- What home treatments is undertaken?

- Was there any additional stress when the pain began?
- Is there any other health problems?
- What kind of work does the patient do?
- Types of recreational activities in which the patient participates

Next, the doctor will make a clinical/physical examination. During the exam, **the doctor may perform any of the following:**

- observe the muscles and joints
- ask to sit and lie down
- ask to move the back in different positions
- observe the most painful area
- check if other areas of the body are tender or painful (such as the kidneys, intestines, or other organs).

If the doctor can identify the likely cause of the back pain, at this point, no further tests will be needed. If the doctor needs more specific information, the following tests may be advised:

## X-ray

Studies show that in many cases of routine back pain, x -rays may not initially be necessary. However, the signs and symptoms will determine what type of study should be done. In certain cases, x-rays might indicate that the pain is due to:

- injury in one or more of the back bones
- a tumor in the spine
- a deformity in the spine
- ankylosing spondylitis

## CAT Scan (Computerized Axial Tomography)

Only a few people with lower back pain need a CAT scan. If the doctor advises one, a special machine takes an x-ray scan of the area. A computer turns this scan into a three-dimensional view of the back. This helps the doctor see if there is a ruptured disc that can't be seen on regular x-rays; CAT scan also helps in detecting spinal stenosis, tumors and infections of the spinal cord.

## MRI (Magnetic Resonance Imaging)

MRI is another way to make very clear pictures of parts of the spine. The MRI does not use x -rays or radioactive dyes. It can provide clearer pictures of soft tissues such as muscles, cartilage, ligaments, tendons and blood vessels in addition to bone structure. To take a MRI picture, the body must be moved very slowly through a tube in the centre of the machine, which contains very powerful magnets. People, who are claustrophobic or whose bodies contain certain kinds of metal objects, may not be able to tolerate the procedure.

The MRI scanner shows the nerves and disc quite clearly. No special dyes or needles are necessary. The MRI scan is, perhaps, too good at showing the anatomic details of the spine. There is a growing body of evidence that suggests that not all abnormalities that show up on the MRI scan are really the cause of the individual patient's problem related to back pain. Abnormalities, such as bulging discs, show up frequently in normal persons who have never had any problem with their back. Hence, it should be kept in mind that a MRI scan is a great test to show the lumbar spine anatomy and it must be correlated carefully with the symptoms so that the findings aren't blown out of proportion.

## Types of Back Pain

Back pain may be acute (generally severe, but short-lived), subacute or chronic (long-lasting or occurring often).

## Acute Back Pain

- Pain usually lasts from one to seven days.
- Pain may be mild or severe.
- An accident or injury occasionally may cause pain.
- About 80 percent of all back pain are acute.

## Subacute Back Pain

- Pain usually lasts from seven days to seven weeks.
- Pain usually is mild and occasionally severe.
- Pain generally is unrelated to other illness.
- About 10 to 20 percent of all back pain are subacute.

## Chronic Back Pain

- Pain usually lasts more than three months.
- Pain may be mild or severe.
- Pain may be related to other illness or may have no identifiable cause.
- About five to 10 percent of all back pain is chronic.

## Structure of Back

The back is held upright by muscles attached to the backbone. Doctors often refer to the backbone as the spine, spinal column, or backbone and find the discs located between each vertebra. These discs are made of cartilage, which is a soft, elastic material, Discs act as cushions, or shock absorbers. Their main job is to protect the joints from wearing out. Most joints contain a slippery substance called synovial fluid that keeps them moving smoothly.

The spinal cord is very important because it transmits electrical signals between the brain and the nerves in the legs, arms, back and other parts of the body. The spinal cord runs through a hole in each vertebra of the upper and middle parts of the backbone, much like a piece of string through a beaded necklace. The space it runs through is called the spinal canal. At times, a message might pain or discomfort. The pain signal is an important one, because it tells that some part of the body needs attention.

A serious injury to the neck or upper back runs the risk of damaging the spinal cord, causing paralysis of the parts of the body below the injury. It should be noted that the spinal cord is not present in the lower part of the backbone. Here the spinal canal contains a sack of nerves, the cauda equina. The backbone, with all its parts, cannot hold itself upright. It needs strong muscles, tendons, and ligaments for support. Muscles help to move or hold the position. Tendons fasten muscles to bones, and ligaments stretch from one bone to another to hold bones together.

## Myelogram

During a myelogram, a special liquid dye called contrast medium is injected into the spinal canal then X-rays are taken of the area. The contrast medium can make problem areas show up more clearly on the x-ray. A myelogram may be ordered to detect problems such as spinal stenosis or spinal cord tumors. If surgery is being considered, particularly for a person who has had a serious back injury, many neurosurgeons will require a myelogram beforehand.

## Bone Scan

During a bone scan, a very small amount of radioactive liquid is injected into a vein which concentrates in the bones for a short time. A special radioactive detecting machine scans the area of concern to produce a picture. Occasionally bone scans are done to look for damage or tumors in the bones themselves. However, back pain is rarely due to diseases of the bones.

## Electrodiagnostic Studies

Electrodiagnostic studies are used to help confirm the presence of nerve compression in the spine. An electrodiagnostic study consists of two tests. One is an electrical test, which is designed to study nerve conduction. In this test the nerve is given an electrical stimulation, and the speed of the impulse is measured. The other test is a needle test called an electromyogram, or EMG. The purpose of this test is to study the muscles for primary disease or for the effect of nerve compression on the muscle. The compression is especially seen in herniated discs or spinal stenosis.

## Blood Tests

If the doctor orders blood tests, a laboratory technician will carefully draw a small amount of blood from a vein in the arm, which will be tested in the laboratory. Anyone of the following blood tests may be advised:

- erythrocyte sedimentation rate (sed rate)
- haematocrit and haemoglobin
- white blood cell count
- HLA B-27 test
- chemical profile (SMAC)

## Treatment

The treatment of back pain ranges from simple reassurance that nothing is wrong to extremely delicate surgery. Each case is different and treatment must be individualized to meet the circumstances. Treatment falls into two major categories:

- Conservative treatment - which includes exercise, medications, physical therapy and other non-operative therapy.
- Surgical treatment-which includes laminectomy, diskectomy and spinal fusion in selected conditions.

Treatment for any back condition should involve two goals:

- To relieve the immediate problem
- To reduce the risk ofre-injury

Exercise plays an important role in achieving both of these goals.

More than 85 percent of people with lower back pain improve with minimal treatment in a matter of days. However, if back problems persist, doctors generally prescribe one or more of the following treatments. For some back conditions, the doctor may refer the patient to another specialist such as an orthopedist, rheumatologists; physical or occupational therapist, psychologist, psychiatrist or surgeon.

## Rest

The most common treatment doctors recommend for severe back pain is bed rest. Different people require different amounts of rest. Usually, two to three days of staying in bed, except to go to the bathroom, will be enough to ease the back pain. The doctor may be consulted to know if special pillows or devices are necessary to give additional support to the neck, back, or feet.

## Heat and Cold

Many people have found that hot and cold treatments help relieve back pain. It is advisable to try both to find out which of the two works best.

Heat relaxes muscles and soothes painful areas. There are many ways to apply heat. Some people like hot showers or baths, while others prefer using heat lamps, heating pads or warm compresses. For the persons having arthritis, heating the muscles first might make it easier to do back exercises. Care should be taken not to fall asleep while using heat.

Cold has a numbing effect. This often helps relieve pain. One of the following methods may be tried for applying cold:

- an ice bag
- a large ice cube used to massage the area
- frozen package of vegetables (peas work best)
- a commercially made cold pack Be sure not to leave ice on after the skin becomes numb as this could lead to localized frostbite. Persons sensitive to ice or having decreased circulation or sensation should not use cold treatment.

13

# Medication and Surgery of Back Pain

If the back pain is not relieved using other forms of treatment, the doctor may prescribe medication. The choice of medication depends on the back pain. For example, medications called analgesics can relieve pain. Other medications called muscle relaxants can help relax tight muscles. If the back pain is caused by arthritis, the doctor can prescribe medication that reduces inflammation as well as relieve the back pain. The most common medications prescribed are called Nonsteroidal anti-inflammatory drugs (NSAIDs). Aspirin and ibuprofen are NSAIDs. Some other NSAID medicines are also prescribed when needed.

Some medications are highly addictive. Pain medication used for prolonged periods has the potential of leading to addiction. No medication will cure back pain of degenerative origin. Medications are used to control pain, inflammation, muscle spasm, and sleep disturbance. Many physicians feel that narcotic medications should not be used on a continuous basis to treat chronic low back pain. There are certain circumstances where pain management specialists are finding that chronic narcotics will actually benefit certain groups of patients with chronic low back pain, but the majority of low back pain will not require this approach.

If simple measures fail to control the back pain, an

Epidural Steroid Injection (ESI) may be suggested. The epidural steroid injection involves placing a small amount of cortisone into the bony spinal canal. Cortisone is a very powerful anti-inflammatory drug that may bring the inflammation surrounding the nerves under control and ease the pain. The epidural steroid injection is not always successful. These injections are reserved for cases where all other conservative measures have failed or as a last attempt to postpone surgery.

A patient should be well informed about his medication and should clarify all doubts regarding the medicines from the doctor.

## About Medication

- ☞ What will the medication do?
- ☞ How long will it take to show results?
- ☞ What is the name of the medication?
- ☞ Is there a generic brand?
- ☞ Are there any side effects?
- ☞ How should the medication be taken? (i.e. before or after meals, with or without food, etc.)
- ☞ How often the medication is to be taken?
- ☞ What is to be done if the dose is not taken at the specified time?

The doctor should be told about the other medication that has been taken as sometimes certain medications cannot be taken together.

## Surgery

People with sciatica or spinal stenosis often benefit from surgery. A few people with tumors within the spinal canal require it. Other than that, few people with back pain need surgery. Most people can be treated successfully with rest, exercise, and medication. Surgery does not always work for many common kinds of back pain, and it is difficult to know who will be helped and who will not. An orthopedist or neurosurgeon can help to decide if a back operation is necessary. It is always recommended to seek a second opinion.

If surgery is suggested for a problem, the best operation for that specific problem will be suggested. Although back surgery is not so common in India, so many people have back problems at some time in their lives that there are substantial number of back operations done. However, the vast majority of people with back problems never have back surgery and function quite well with a minimal effect on their daily lives. An overview of the general types of back surgery that are sometimes necessary is given below.

One of the most common surgical procedures is a diskectomy, the removal of a herniated disc to relieve pressure on a nerve root. The first step is to remove a portion of the lamina of the vertebra. The lamina is the portion of the vertebra that forms the roof over the spinal nerves. Removing a portion of the lamina creates a window into the spine. The nerves are then pulled to the side so that the herniated disc can be seen. Small instruments are then used to remove the herniated disc material. Most of the nucleus pulposus is removed to prevent the disc from herniating again. Once the disc material is removed, the nerves are free of pressure and irritation. The lamina and the area of the disc that is removed fill with scar tissue very rapidly.

When the major problem appears to be spinal stenosis the spinal canal needs to be made larger. This is done by performing a complete laminectomy. The lamina is the backportion of the spine and forms the roof of the spinal canal. The term laminectomy means to remove the lamina. Removal of lamina allows more room for the nerves and enables the surgeon to remove bone spurs around the nerves. This allows more room for the nerves of the spine and reduces the irritation and inflammation on the spinal nerves. The bone does not grow back. Instead, scar tissue replaces the lamina and protects the spinal nerves.

If the back problem is the result of segmental instability, a spinal fusion may be suggested. A spinal fusion involves placing a bone graft between two or more vertebrae, causing the vertebrae to grow together or fuse. The bone graft is usually taken from the bones of the pelvis at the time of surgery. There are two general types of spinal fusion:

- ☞ Posterior fusion
- ☞ Interbody fusion

In the posterior fusion, the bone graft is placed on the back side of the vertebrae. During the healing process the vertebrae then fuse, or grow together. This creates a solid block of bone between the vertebrae, and the vertebra that is fused together act like one bone. The Interbody fusion differs by placing the bone graft between the vertebrae, where the disc has been removed. Once again, the healing process causes the vertelirae to fuse, creating a solid block of bone between the fused vertebrae. Both fusions accomplish the same thing. The vertebrae grow together, or fuse into one bone. The goal of a spinal fusion is to stop the motion between two vertebrae that comes from segmental instability. Fusing the vertebrae together reduces the mechanical back pain and impingement on the nerve root that comes from too much motion between the vertebrae.

14

# Backache: Top 10 Treatments Revealed

## A Cute Pain

1. Take over the counter painkillers. But be cautious. A recent study found that regular use of common pain relievers such as Ibuprofen may cause high blood pressure.
2. See an osteopath or chiropractor for manipulation of the spine and exercises. You will require between two and six sessions.
3. Try acupuncture, in which very thin needless are inserted under the skin.
   Pain relief can result from the release of endorphins, the body's own pain relieving chemicals.

## Moderate to Severe Pain

4. See your GP, who may prescribe stronger anti inflammatory pain killers than can be bought over the counter.
   Nonsteroid anti-inflammatories can have side effects, including ulcers.
5. Your GP may also prescribe a muscle relaxant such as diazepam, to be taken for a short period to reduce muscle spasms.
6. Have physiotherapy. A physiotherapist can design

an exercise programme to improve your flexibility, strengthen your back and improve your posture.

7. Take oral steroids, which may be prescribed during episodes of pain. These reduce inflammation in the spine. Oral steroids are intended for use for short periods of time
8. Have steroid injections, which can reduce pain and inflammation.
9. Have an epidural. Corticosteroid drugs can be injected into the spine and are used in the treatment of sciatica. The effects will last a few months.
10. Have surgery- usually the last resort and only in the most severe cases. Back operations include spinal fusion and the removal of disc material that is compressing nerves.

## Novel spinal surgery

Scientists in the US are using a novel technique to remove tumours from the cervical region of the spine that were previously thought inoperable, according to a study published in operative Neurosurgery.

Called a lateral paramedian transpedicular approach, the technique uses standard and innovative devices to first remove and then reconstruct portions of the cervical spine.

Once the bone is removed, surgeons have a direct line of sight to the tumour and can remove it in entirety without a touch to the spinal cord.

# 15

# PROPER EXERCISES & POSTURES FOR BACKACHE

For many people, the key to a healthy back is proper exercise. Some exercises are designed to strengthen the back and stomach muscles, while other exercises are designed to improve the posture. A 30-minute aerobic program, three times a week, is ideal for overall fitness. Walking and! or water exercises are highly recommended for most people with back problems. The right kind of exercise program may help keep the back problem under control. It makes easy to continue the daily activities.

In the early stages, when the back is still quite painful, the specific exercises, which reduce the pain are advised. These exercises are helpful in easing pain through relaxation. The positioning exercises help in placing the spine at a resting position. These exercises give relief to sore muscles and joints.

Movement is also important, even when the back is still painful. The therapists suggest careful movements that can safely ease pain by providing nutrition and lubrication to injured areas. Movement of joints and muscles also signals the nervous system to block incoming pain. As the back becomes less painful, the exercises will be changed to focus on improving the overall health of the back. These changes will focus on:

- flexibility
- strength
- coordination

- aerobic conditioning

Exercises help in reducing pain and to keep the spine in the neutral position. Tight muscles can cause an imbalance in spinal movements and make the risk of injury to these structures more likely. Flexibility exercises for the trunk and lower limbs are helpful in establishing a pattern of safe movement. The stretching exercises also increase the flexibility in the muscles and ligaments of the back and reduce the chance of re-injury.

The next stage of exercise focuses on the strength of the muscles that support the spine. These muscles help bring the spine into the normal shape. Well-trained abdominal, back and hip muscles can help hold the back in a neutral position, almost forming a natural corset. Strength training is simple to do at home and doesn't require any expensive equipment.

Posture exercises help train the muscles in the right movements between the pelvis and low back. Learning how to find and hold the neutral position of the spine - is the key for a safe and healthy posture. It should always be kept in mind that the position of the pelvis determines the curve in the low back. Forward rotation increases the curve while the backward rotation straightens the curve. By practicing these exercises one will become more comfortable in using the neutral spine position in the daily activities. Strong muscles need to be coordinated. As the strength of the spinal muscle increases, it becomes important to train those muscles to work together.

Learning any physical activity requires practice. Muscles must be trained so that the physical activity should always remain under control. Muscles trained to control safe movement of the spine reduce the chance of injury. There are certain exercises that train the back muscles to work together to protect the spine.

Finally, attention will be directed to increase the overall fitness. Muscles get the energy they need to work either by using oxygen to bum calories from the bloodstream or by burning sugars in the bloodstream quickly without using oxygen. By using oxygen, muscles are better able to move continuously, rather than in spurts. The word aerobic means intake of lot of oxygen. Fitness training, or aerobic training, conditions the muscles to become better able to obtain the nutrients and oxygen that they need from the blood. If muscles are more used to working in fits and spurts they are more likely to bum sugars without using oxygen. This is called anaerobic metabolism, and it doesn't work nearly as well as aerobic metabolism. As the muscles use up the nutrients and oxygen, they switch to anaerobic metabolism and chemical waste products are created that can cause pain in the muscles. Aerobic training increases the muscles ability to get rid of these waste products.

Exercise has other benefits as well. Exercise can cause chemicals called endorphins to be released into the blood. These chemical hormones act as natural pain relievers in reducing the pain. So, exercise can actually help control pain through the body's natural pain medication. It will be important to pick up an aerobic activity that is enjoyable and can be stuck to. But the exercise that makes the back pain worse should be avoided. The doctor or physical therapist may be consulted to know the right exercises.

## Maintaining Good Posture

Mother Nature did not design the human spine to sit. Sitting, and especially sitting for long periods of time, is a lot harder on the back than lying down, standing up and even lifting (assuming that lifting is done properly).

This has something to do with what happens to the spine when the posture is changed from standing to sitting. The lower back has a natural curve called a lordotic curve. It's important to maintain natural lordosis. In this position, the structures that support the spine-the muscles, ligaments and discs can work in harmony.

If the back is not supported, the muscles will get very tired, very quickly. When this happens, the body slouches in an attempt to give those muscles a rest. The problem is that sitting in a slouched posture reduces the natured lumbar curve. That's one of the main reasons why so many people's discs bulge and/or herniate.

By sitting properly in an ergonomically designed chair, the back will be supported correctly. But this may not be enough, as backs are not built to sit in the same position for long periods of time, even when the posture is perfect. Hence it is very important to practise techniques for good posture while sitting, standing or sleeping.

## When Sitting

- Sit in a firm chair with armrests to relieve pressure in the back and shoulders.
- Keep the upper back straight and shoulders relaxed. Keep stomach muscles pulled in and maintain the proper curve in the lower back. Tightening the stomach and buttocks can do this. Some people are more comfortable sitting with the back of the chair at a 15- to 20-degree angle. A small cushion behind the lower back to maintain the natural curve of the back also can be quite helpful.
- Keep the knees slightly higher than the hips. Use a footstool or book under the feet if necessary.
- Keep the feet flat on the floor or other surface.
- Don't sit for a long period of time. Stand up every now and then so as to stretch tight muscles and give them a chance to relax.

## When Standing

- Stand with weight equal on both feet.
- Avoid locking the knees.
- Ease tension in the back by placing one foot on a footstool.
- Those who stand for long periods of time should wear flat or low-heeled shoes.
- Keep the back straight by tightening the stomach muscles and buttocks.

## When Sleeping

- Lie on the side with the knees bent.
- If feel more comfortable, place a pillow between the knees while sleeping on the side.
- If one sleeps on the back, ask the doctor or physical therapist if placing pillows under the knees would help the lower back pain or make it worse.
- Use a hard mattress.

## Body Mechanics

Good body mechanics mean to keep good posture while in motion. For example, while lifting, the object lifted is to be held close to the body and lifting should be done with the weight on legs. Thus the normal back curves are maintained as the legs lift the load. Avoidance of twisting, particularly when carrying a load, is also important for good body mechanics.

- When bending down to lift an object, bend with the knees instead of the back.
- Hold the object close to you.
- Straighten the legs to lift the object.
- Get help with an object that is too heavy.

The type of shoes also affects the posture. High heels

may put more stress on the lower back by changing the posture. It is more comfortable to wear low or flat heels. Cushion-soled shoes also provide "shock absorbency" for the spine.

### Weight Loss

One way of reducing the back pain and improving the general health is to lose weight, preferably with a balanced diet along with regular exercise. Fad diets or fast weight-loss programs are to be avoided. These can be harmful and may cause new problems.

16

# PAIN IN THE NECK

We've all scoffed at that 'pain in the neck'. But watch out for that, especially after an accident-it could be a block in the neck artery and harbinger of a stroke. Clots cause 70-80% of all strokes and can cause paralysis and death in extreme cases.

Rahul Sharma, a 27 year old, was lucky. He was speeding in his car with a friend when severe pain hit the left side of his neck. Before his friend could react, Rahul slumped in his seat, unconscious. He was rushed to hospital where doctors gave him blood thinners to prevent further complications.

"This block in the neck artery," says Dr. V. K. Dixit, consultant, interventional neuro radiologist, VIMHANS, "usually happens during severe accidents or while doing head stands. The young are more susceptible to it due to their love of speed." Although any artery in the neck may be affected, internal carotid artery blockages are the most common.

Arteries are made of layers. Blockages generally occur between the first and second layers of an artery, says Dr Harsh Rastogi, interventional neuro radiologist, Apollo Hospital. "During an injury, there is a rent in the inner fragile layer of the artery. Blood with higher BP will rush in, making the vessel narrow and decreasing blood flow to brain. Before a full block occurs, this has to be treated with angioplasty and stenting to restore blood supply," he asserts.

The symptoms of a block include a "thunderclap" headache never experienced before, neck pain, vomiting and episodic blindness caused by decreased blood flow to the retina. "Usually the pain becomes severe over time," says Rastogi. "There might be loss of consciousness for a few seconds or sudden weakness which progresses over time, dizziness which does not respond to the usual medication, weakness in limbs and coma. These need urgent attention before a transient stroke occurs."

Studies have found that approximately 20% of strokes in the young are caused by carotid and vertebral artery blockages in the neck, compared to 2.5% in older patients. Annual incidence of carotid artery blockage in US is 2.6 per lakh population. In India, it's about 7-10 cases a month in any big hospital; 90% are trauma patients.

Dixit also warns of transient ischemic attacks (TIA)- temporary strokeswhere the patient recovers within 24 hours. Warning symptoms are weakness in one half of the body, temporary loss of speech and blurring of vision." Just like an angina is an indication of heart attack, these are in dictions of a stroke coming on, " he says.

Angioplasty reinforced with a stent can prevent a stroke from occurring. Here's how it works. Stents are compressed into a catheter. Using X-rays, an interventional neuro radiologist inserts the catheter through an incision in the groin. It's advanced through the femoral artery to tiny arteries where the clot busting drug is delivered directly into the hardened artery to break the clot.

The procedure costs between Rs. 1.5-2 lakh and the patient can often resume normal life with minimal or no after effects, say doctors.

# 17

# Massage Step-by-step For Relief Of Pain In Different Organs

Just before you begin your massage check that your hands and clean and your nails fairly short with no jagged edges. Take off any rings if you wear them. You will find if you use aromatherapy oils regularly that your nails strengthen and your hands become smoother and more supple. Also, check with your massage partner to make sure there are no reasons to stop you going ahead.

## The Feet

Probably the most neglected part of our bodies, feet deserve a loving massage from time to time. Make sure your partner is warm and comfortable. Uncover one foot by folding back the towel or blanker. Now pour a little of your chosen oil into the palm of one hand. Rub your hands together to evenly distribute the oil. Now you are ready to begin.

1. Enclose the foot between both hands (one on top, one underneath), then gently slide your hands off the foot coming forward to the toes. This movement should be slow and soothing. Repeat four or five times.
2. Gently circle around the ankles using your thumbs. This area can be tender, so go easy.
3. Rub over the top of the foot with your thumbs

in little circles, coming down from the andkle area to the toes. Repeat three or four times.

4. Now rub each toe with the same little circular movements.
5. Rotate each toe twice in each direction.
6. Gently pull each toe between finger and thumb.
7. Zigzag down the sole of the foot from toes to heel with your thumbs overlapped.
8. Enclose the foot in your hands then rub them in opposite directions, to create frictions. This is very warming.
9. Hold the foot firmly and slowly rotate the ankle clockwise then anti-clockwise. Repeat a couple of times.
10. Repeat step 1.

Once complete, wrap the foot up again for warmth and repeat the movements on the repeat the movements on the other foot. By now your massage partner will be feeling more relaxed and at ease with your touch.

## The Lower Legs And Knees

Warm a little oil in your hands.

1. With one hand behind the other, smooth the oil on to the front of the leg, starting at the top of the foot and working up to the knee. This movement distributes the oil and soothes and relaxes the whole area.
2. Rub acroos the front of the leg using both hands to create frictions. This increases the blood circulation to the area and reduces aches and pains.
3. Lift the leg up so the knee is bent. Squeeze and relax rhythmically down the muscles of the calf from knee to ankle. Repeat several times. Put the leg down.
4. Work around the kneecap in little circular motions with both hands. Be careful not to use too much

pressure.

5. Now using your thumbs gently slide them around each side of the kneecap.
6. Stretch out your thumbs from your fingers to create an arch. Sweep over the whole knee using alternate hands several times.

Now Wrap up the lower leg and proceed to the thigh.

## The Upper Legs

1. Apply oul as for trhe lower leg.
2. Glide up the leg from knee to groin, using one hand behind the other. This movement should be fairly slow and rhythmical. Make sure your movements cover the whole of the thigh area. Repeat four to five times.
3. Stroke the upper inner thigh diagonally from knee to groin hand over hand. Repeat four or five times.
4. Squeeze and release rhythmically first along the inner thigh from knee to groin, then along the outer thigh.
5. Using your knuckles rake quickly up from the knee to the groin, taking in the whole thigh area. This is a friction movement and increases the surface blood circulation. You'll notice the skin colours quite quickly and feels warmer to the touch.
6. Uncover the lower leg, then effleurage the whole leg from foot to groin as in step 2.
7. Finish off by enclosing the foot in your hands a couple of times. Cover the leg then repeat all the movements on the other one.

By now you'll find your hands have become more sensitive to your partner and you'll notice differences in the skin texture and muscle tone.

## The Hands and Arms

1. Smooth on the oil as before. When working on the arm it's easier to effleurage with one hand only, using the other to hold the arm steady.
2. Bend the arm at the elbow. Massage around the wrist with little thumb circles using both hands.
3. Work down from the wrist to the ends of the fingers using little thumb circles. Repeat five times.
4. Stretch each finger, then thumb, in turn between your finger and thumb.
5. Rotate the fingers and thumb first clockwise then anti-clockwise.
6. Turn the hand over and rub gently along the solar plexus (from centre wrist down the palm to the middle finger) using alternate thumbs. This is calming to the nervours system.
7. Rotate the hand at the wrist clockwise then anti-clockwise. To do this lock your fingers into your partner's.
8. Turn the hand over and work on the insode of the wrist up to the elbow using alternate sweeping movements. Repeat four or five times.
9. Bend the arm at the elbow and bring the lower arm up and across the chest. Squeeze all along the upper arm from elbow to shoulder using both hands.
10. Bring the arm back down to the side then effleurage the whole area from hand to shoulder four or five times. Cover the arm and repeat on the other side.

## The Abdomen

The abdomen is a soft area protecting vital organs, so please be gentle. Fold the towel or blanket down to expose the area from just below the breasts to a couple of inches (centimetres) below the navel.

1. Apply oil, starting just under the rib-cage, working down and out towards the waist. Be careful to keep your hands relaxed and contoured to your partner. Poking fingers feel very uncomfortable here.
2. With one hand on top of the other iron around the lower abdomen in large circles. Keep the pressure light and even.
3. Fan your hands out and work from the navel out to the waist. Slide your hands under the waist then gently pull them back round to the front again. Repeat several times.
4. Stroke diagonally with alternate hands from the waist down to below the navel, first on the left side, then on the right.
5. Stroke down from the solar plexus to the navel, one hand behind the other, to finish off this area.

## The Backs of The legs

1. Effleurage oil as for the front of the legs but working from the foot right up to the top of the thigh. Repeat four of five times.
2. Bend the leg at the knee, supporting it with one hand. Stroke firmly down the calf, across behind the knee, then back up to the foot several times keeping your hands contoured to the leg. Put the leg down.
3. Work up the calf to the knee, using little circles. Repeat several times to cover the whole calf.
4. Using your index and middle fingers, make small circular movements behind the knee. Be careful not to press too hard.
5. Squeeze rhythmically along the inner thigh from

the knee upwards. Repeat on the outer thigh, doing each movement several times.

6. Diagonally stroke from the inner knee upwards and across the thigh. Repeat several times.
7. Finish by effeuraging the whole leg several times, from foot to thigh. Wrap up and repeat on the other leg.

## The Back

Don't be at all surprised if your massage partner dozes off at this point. Back massage is extremely soothing and relaxing and great for relieving stress and tension.

Uncover the back to just show the buttock crease. At this point it is a good idea to place a small rolled-up towel under your partner's forehead otherwise he or she will have to turn his or her head sideways or end up with a squashed nose through which it is difficult to breathe.

1. Starting at the lower back effleurage oil using both hands. Work slowly up the back to the shoulders, pressing gently on the upward strokes, releasing the pressure as you come back down.
2. Starting at the base of the spine work up on either side, using gentle thumb pressure or little thumb circles. Repeat five or six times.
3. With reinforced hands (one on top of the other) sweep up the spine then work around the shoulder blades in a figure-of-eight movement. Repeat the figure-of-eight four or five times.
4. Now work around each shoulder blade individually, still with reinforced hands, in a circular motion. Repeat four of five times each side. You may feel knots (little bumps) around the shoulder blades. These are an indication of tension, and massage here gives great relief.
5. Work around the shoulder blades with your

thumbs, helping to break down the knots and bumps. Allow your partner to be your guide as these areas can be tender.

6. Squeeze along the top of the shoulders from the neck out, using your fingers and thumbs. Repeat four to five times on each side.
7. Stroke up the back of the neck and out to the ears, using your thumbs.
8. Stand at your partner's head and sweep your hands down the centre back, across the top of the buttocks, then firmly pull up at the sides. Repeat five times.
9. Move to your partner's side and rub backwards and forwards over the whole back with frictions to warm the area.
10. Make thumb circles out from just above the buttock crease round towards the hips. This area can often be tender and massage here is soothing. Repeat several times.
11. Effleurage the whole back.
12. Gently stroke up the spine, hand over hand, several times, allowing your touch to get lighter and lighter.
13. Finish by gently holding your partner. Place one hand at the base of the spine, the other at the base of the neck. Hold this position and feel the warmth build up under your hands. After approximately one minute gently lift your hands off. Cover your partner over.

    By now, he or she might be snoozing!

## The Shoulders and Neck

If your partner is feeling very tense, and you haven't time to give a full body massage, working on the shoulders and neck will still offer great relief. For this your partner should be lying on his or her back. Uncover the chest by folding down the towel or blanket.

1. Apply oil to your partner's chest, shoulders and neck.
2. Begin effleuraging by placing both hands on the upper chest, fingers facing towards each other. Now, slowly pull your hands across the chest and out to the shoulders. Curve your hands round the shoulders and under them, then bring your hands in to meet at the back of the neck. Stroke up the neck to the base of the skull, Repeat four or five times.
3. Gently knuckle the chest and shoulders in the sequence shown in the diagram on the left. To knuckle make your hands into relaxed fists, and move the knuckles in circular movements. This sounds more difficult than it is.
4. Gently turn your partner's head to one side. Stroke along the top of the shoulder and the side of the neck with your first three fingers. Repeat three times.
5. Repeat the above sequence, but circle your fingers this time. Do this three times.
6. Turn your partner's head to the other side and repeat movements 4 and 5. Return the head to the centre.
7. Slide your hands down your partner's back as far as you can comfortably reach. Find the groove each side of the spine with your fingers. Pull your hands up the spine with a little pressure on the groove each side. Repeat three times.
8. Now you are going to stretch the neck - these movements stretch out the muscles of the shoudlers and ncek and ease tension. If your partner is relaxed you'll find you will take all the weight of the head. If he or she is tense, go easy and

make the movements slow and gentle. You don't want any pulled muscles.

9. Cup both hands unde your partner's head, your fingers resting in the base of the skull. Lift the head slightly, then gently pull towards you. Lower the head slowly, then repeat.
10. Hold the back of the head in one hand and move it slowly towards the left shoulder while gently pressing down on the right shoulder with your other hand. Bring the head back to the centre and then repeat on the other side.
11. Finish with some effleurage movements as you begin.

## The Face And Scal

Until you've had the pleasurable experience of a face massage you probably won't have realized how much tension we hold in our faces. Think of frowning - this is caused by muscle action, and these muscles tire just as much as those of any other part of the body. A caring face massage can smooth away some of this tension, leaving us looking (and feeling) more at ease and relaxed.

Offer to take your partner's hair off the face with a headband, as it will inevitably get a little ouly around the hairline during the massage. Be careful not to use too much oil on the face or you'll find it difficult to massage specific areas without slipping.

Encourage your partner to close his or her eyes, so as to focus on your touch. Also, it can be disconcerting to have someone staring up at you, especially as a novice.

1. Begin by stroking up each side of the jawline to the forehead. Repeat four or five times.
2. Slowly stroke the forehead rhythmically with the flat of your hand from just above the brows to the hairline.

3. Starting at the centre hairline slide your thumbs out to the side, applying gentle pressure. Move down the forehead slightly and repeat. Continue this outward stroking pressure until you reach the eyebrows.
4. Now place the heel of each hand on the centre forehead and slide out to the sides. Repeat three times.
5. Place the first two fingers of each hand on the temples and circle gently for a minute or two, applying a little pressure.

   All the above movements help to relieve a headache. Try lavender oil for yourmassage, as I've found it can ward off a headache if used in time.
6. Place your thumbs on your partner's inner eyebrows and slide out to the sides. Repeat three times.
7. With your index finger and thumb gently pull along the brow bone. Repeat three times.
8. Stroke gently over the eyelids with your ring fingers, from the inner to the outer conrners. Repeat three times.
9. Alternately stroke down the nose with your thumbs, then gently rub round the nose tip and nostrils. Be careful not to press hard on the nostrils.
10. Stroke the cheeks across the cheekbones and gradually work down the face to the chin.
11. Make little circular movements across the top lip. When you reach the corner of the mouth lift slightly, then repeat.
12. Make pinching movements out along the jawline and up towards the ears.
13. Rub the earlobes between your fingers and thumb, then gently pinch all around the outer ear. Most people love this.
14. Sweep your hands up the neck and on to the

cheeks. Hold, then repeat.

15. Finish by stroking the forehead, getting lighter and lighter until you bring your hands off.

## Scalp Movements

1. Remove your partner's headband. Bring your hands up the side of the face to the forehead, then rake them through the hair. Repeat several times.
2. 'Glue' your fingers onto the scalp and move it around against the skull. Move your fingers to a different position and repeat this process until all the scalp has been covered.
3. Rub vigorously over the scalp, as if shampooing the hair.
4. Take little bunches of hair all over the scalp and tug gently. This feels lovely and really stimulates the scalp.
5. Repeat step 1 to finish off.

18

# YOGIC KRIYAS TO DETOXIFY THE BODY AND RELIEVE PAIN

These Yogic Kriyas are the purification processes of the body by yogic methods. They are very important in Yoga. Union of body with mind, union of mind with soul and union of soul with God is Yoga.

Kriyas are to be practised early in the morning before rise on empty stomach. Kriyas must be finished before starting the Asanas or Pranayama.

Among these kriyas only Kapalbhati is not related to water. All other five kriyas are water related and helpful in eliminating several disorders.

These Kriyas consist of six purification practises -

1. Dhauti (Kunjal)
2. Basti
3. Neti
4. Tratak
5. Nauli, and
6. Kapalbhati.

## Dhauti (Kunjal)

Vomit-Dhauti-Cleaning. Washing stomach by water.

Two or three litre of tepid water is required. Squat on your feet back, spine and neck should be straight. Drink glasses of tepid water continuously without any pause upto the brim of neck. One should neither talk nor laugh during this period. He should not bend and should stand.

Bend a bit forward. Keep the left hand on the left knee and the first and second finger of the right hand in your throat. Press the stomach by the other hand. You will vomit. Vomit the whole drunk water. Water should not remain in stomach.

Wash you hands and take rest. Milk or breakfast should be taken after an hour.

This Dhauti kriya should be practised after passing stool and after bath. One should not take bath after this kriya. Vaman Dhauti kriya should be practised once a fortnight or once a month.

Precautions - 1. Heart patients should not practise it. 2. The nails of the fingers should be trimmed otherwise they may wound the throat.

Benefits - 1. Disorders of bile and gas are cured. 2. It is beneficial in the diseases of stomach throat and jaundice.

## Basti (Enema)

Enema pot, rubber tube, nozzle, tepid water, lemon are the requirements. Mix juice of one or two lemons in the tepid water. Fill the enema pot with water.

Suspend the enema pot one metre above. Apply a little oil or vaseline to the nozzle of the rectal tube. Before insertion, check the rectal tube to ensure free flow of water. Insert the tube into the rectum. The flow of water can be adjusted with the knob attached to the tube. When all the water has been introduced, remove the tube and resist the pressure for a few minutes. The bowels can be emptied after a while for better cleansing. If one does not wish to take enema in the lying position he can take it in the standing position.

*Special note* - Enema should be taken after going to latrine. Salt can be mixed in water instead of lemon juice. You can use plain water also. Soap should not be mixed in water.

## Precautions

1. Enema should be taken once in a week or in a month by a healthy person.
2. It can be taken for two to four days daily in constipation.
3. Take rest for half an hour after enema.
4. Do not take any thing after enema for an hour.

## Benefits

1. Removes constipation.
2. Cleans bowels.
3. Beneficial in all diseases of stomach.

## Neti

It is mainly of two types:
i. Jala Neti    ii. Sutra Neti.

## Jala Neti

For doing this, squat on your feet. Take tepid salted water in a medium sized pot with along spout, made especially for this purpose.

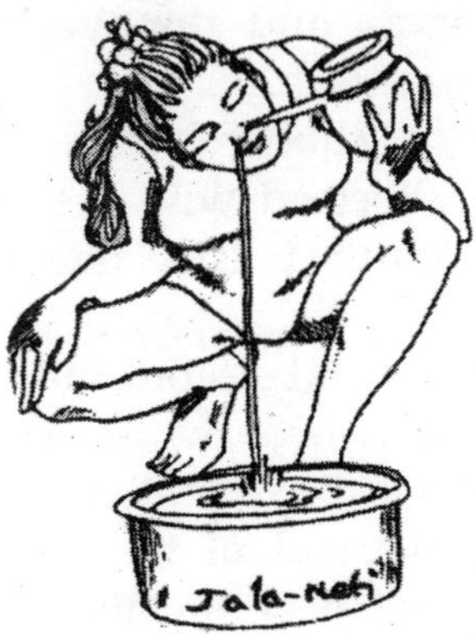

Now fill the pot with tepid salted water and hold it in your right hand to the level of your nose. Then tilt your head slightly to the left so as to have the slanting position of the left nostril. Insert the nozzle of the spout into the right nostril and allow the water to flow down slowly. The water should continue falling down from other nostril in a continuous thin stream. Now repeat the process from the other side. Breath through the mouth only till the kriya is complete. After Jal Neti, stand erect with your feet together. Keep the hands behind your back clasped and blow out vigorously whatever trace of water that has remained in your nostrils.

*Precautions* - If sometimes one feels intolerable pain in the back of ear or above nostrils, he should practise the Kriya of Kapalbahit at once. It will cure the pain.

Water can come out of eyes in beginning of Neti. These can be warmed. Do not fear.

## Benefits

- It cures sinusitis and clears sinuses.
- It cures diseases of nose, eyes, throat and prevents the occurrence of diseases.
- It purifies mind.
- It improves memory.
- It cures coryza and removes old accumulated phlegm.

Sutra Neti or Rubber Neti

Sutra Neti is performed with a 12 inches long piece of waxed cord. It is partly twisted and it makes the nasal insertion possible.

Squat on your feet. Take tepid salted water and soak the Neti well in it. Now take the waxed and twisted end of the cord and make it to curve. Bend your head slightly forward and insert the end of the cord into the nostril through which you have been breathing at that time. Push the cord gradually through the nose, down the throat. Now open your mouth wide, put your index and middle fingers in and with their tips catch the inside end of the cord and draw it out. Hold both the ends in you hand separately and pull the cord very gently up and down three to four times. Then take it out, wash it and then repeat the cycle with the other nostril.

After completion of the kriya, wash the cord with soap well and leave it to dry in some clean and safe place so that the flies, etc. do not pollute it.

## Special note

- When the cord reaches throat through nostrils, it becomes greasy by mucurs. Therefore, both the ends of the cord should be caught firmly.
- Sutra Neti or Rubber Neti should be practised after learning Jal Neti. After this one can practise Neti with milk, oil or ghee.
- It is more beneficial to perform this Sutra Neti by cotton cord but it should be wrapped.

## Precautions

- One can sneeze in practising Sutra Neti. Water can come out of eyes. One should not fear. Practise makes one perfect.
- Nose can bleed sometimes while performing Sutra Neti. In such conditions use rubber catheter (No. 4) instead of cotton cord. Move the cord through nostrils and throat slowly and gently.

## Benefits

- It cures all diseases of nose.
- It reduces polyp in nose.

- It cures sinusitis.
- It cures coryza.
- It improves eyesight.
- It improves memory.
- It purifies mind.

## Nasapan

Drinking water through nostrils is called nasapan. One should clean the nostrils before drinking water through them.

## Milk Neti

Milk is used in place of water. Milk should be without malai cream.

*Benefits*-Nasapan prevents cold and coryza. It improves eyesight.

## Oil Neti

Mustard oil should be made warm in a spoon. When it is lukewarm and tolerable to the skin, lie down on a bed and drip five or seven drops of oil through some dropper in both the nostrils and try to draw them in. You will feel that the oil going in. You can use clean cotton instead of Dropper. Coconut or almond oil can be used in place of mustard of. Pure ghee can also be used. Three or four drops of ghee or Bhadan Ragan are sufficient for the nostrils.

Oil Neti or Neti of ghee should be done before going to bed at night.

*Benefits*-It lubricates noses and cleanses it. It prevents from cold and coryza.

## Tratak

It is an amazing exercise to improve your power of concentration, eyesight and pain of eye nuycles.

It can be practised with a candle or with a black dot on a piece of paper fixed on the wall. Start this practice in a closed room, as there will be less objects to disturb your concentration.

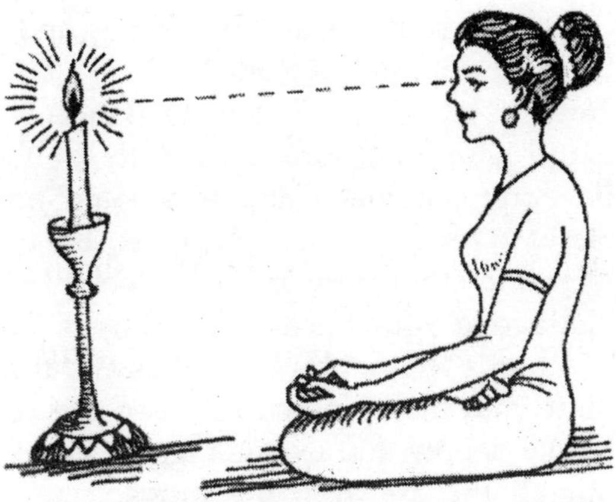

Sit on floor in any comfortable of Padmasana pose. Keep your back and spinal cord erect. Have a few deep breaths. Make your breath steady, even and rhythmic. Keep the object of your gaze at your eye level at a distance of three to four feet. Keep the eyes meditatively wide out of your eyes. Close the eyes to let tears trickle down.

Now mentally visualize that object when the mental image visualizes, open your eyes and start gazing afresh. Do not strain your nerves and get relaxed. Let not your mind wander. Try to bring your mind back to the object but without straining yourself much as that would sap your energy and you will be tired soon.

After practising with the point on the walls or on a steady flame, try to-do it concentrating on the tip of your nose on the point between the eyebrows.

## Benefits

1. Tartar improves eyesight and removes the diseases of eyes.
2. It helps in concentrating your mind.
3. It purifies your mind.

## Nauli Kriya

It is the best exercise for preserving and promoting the health of abdominal viscera.

- Nauli is equal to Uddiyana Bandh.
- Nauli should be practised daily in the morning on empty stomach and evacuated bowels.
- Stand with legs one foot apart. Bend the legs a little and stoop forward. Rest the palms on thighs just above your knees, with fingers spread. Press the thighs well with your palms and the chest with your chin at the notch between the collar bones.
- Inhale deeply and exhale vigorously so as to force out all the air from the lungs.
- Suspend the breath and pull the abdominal region back towards the spine so that a hollow is formed.
- Push the abdominal recti forward so that a vertical ridge down the centre is formed. remain in this position for a few seconds and then relax the gap and inhale smoothly.
- Breath deeply three to four times and then repeat the cycle. Repeat it five to seven times.

## Special note

1. Nauli kriya is not easy. Obese persons feel difficulty in its practise. It is essential to practice Uddiyana Bandh and Agnisar to perform Nauli.
2. Nauli kriya should be performed on empty

stomach after cleaning bowels and before taking food.

3. One should wear only underwear while practising Nauli. Women can wear bra/ brassiere also.

## Precautions

1. Nauli should be practised on empty stomach.
2. It should not be practised unless there is some expert to demonstrate and then to guide and supervise the whole process.
3. It should not be practised before the age of 12 or 13 years.
4. The ulcer patient and the weak person should perform Nauli on the advice of Yoga therapist.
5. The patients suffering from swelling of intestines, dysentery, hernia and high blood pressure should not practice Nauli.

*Benefits*-The benefits of Nauli are many. It strengthens the abdominal muscles and liver. Women who suffer from a menstrual problem get immediate relief. It increases gastric fire and helps eliminating the toxic elements from the digestive system. It also helps in ovarian insufficiency. Nauli quickly cures constipation, dyspepsia, flatulence etc.

## Kapalbhati

Kapal means skull. Bhati means shine or lustre, Thus, this term means "skull shining". Kapalbhati is a Pranayama also besides one of the six cleaning exercises. Actually this kriya or cleansing process is a milder form of Bhastrika, another vigorously breathing exercise.

Sit on a blanket or a dari in Padmasana, Sidhasana or Sukhasana. Keep back, spinal cord and neck erect. Keep both the hands on knees. Shut your eyes. Sit peacefully.

Exhale vigorously. Do not inhale. At start begin slowly after four to five exhales exhale vigorously and quickly. Be careful in exhaling; you will inhale between exhales.

One should not pause during the practice of Kapabhati. Hold the breath after exhaling (Kumbhak). During Kumbhak practice Jallandhar Bandh, Uddiyana Bandh, Mool Bandh and Mahabandh. Hold this position for a while. Release all Bandhs and inhale slowly. This completes one round of Kapalbhati. Start with two rounds. You can practice unto five rounds gradually. Start with ten or twelve exhales. Gradually you can increase their number 50 to 120.

## Special Note

1. The stomach should go inside at once after exhaling.
2. The difference between Kapabhati and Bhasrika Pranayam is that both inhale and exhale are done vigorously. One should learn it from an expert in Yogic Kriya.

*Precautions*-Persons with high BP problems or pus in the ear should refrain from doing this exercise.

*Benefits*-This Kapalbhati is very good invigorating exercise which cleanses the entire respiratory system by forcefully rushing exhalation.

It removes concentration and mental retention. The movement of the diaphragm stimulates the stomach, heart liver and spleen. This exercise is very good for eyes.

## Agnisar

The practice of Agnisar kindles energy in stomach and body perspires.

Sit on a blanket or dari in Vajrasana. Keep a little distance between the knees. Put firmly both the hands on the knees. Inhale vigorously and while exhaling shrink your stomach as much as you can. Now suspend your breath. It is called Bahya Kumbhak.

Holding the position of Bahya Kumbhak, i.e. Keeping the breath suspended and pulling the entire abdominal region back towards your spine. Now blow your stomach out and shrink in . In one Kumbhak you can blow and shrink your stomach 8-20 times .

This kriya is called Agnisar. One can practice this kriya in a standing posture.

## Benefits

1. Cures obesity.
2. Cures disorders of abdominal region.
3. It improves lack of appetite.

## Bandh

Bandh means binding. Bandhs literally means a lock, bondage or joining together to objects or stages. A Bandh is a special posture invented to conserve and make greater use of vast resources of energy generated by yogic exercises and Pranayama. These Bandhs are means of reorientation and control of the vital energy of your body and mind. These are of three main types.

## Jalandhar Bandh

It this Bandh the throat is contracted blocked, as it were, by making the chin rest on the chest in the notch between the collar bones in certain asanas or posture like Sarvangasana exhalation and fresh, when the breath is suspended. Once in a day early in the morning it should be practised, first standing, then in advanced stage in the sitting position.

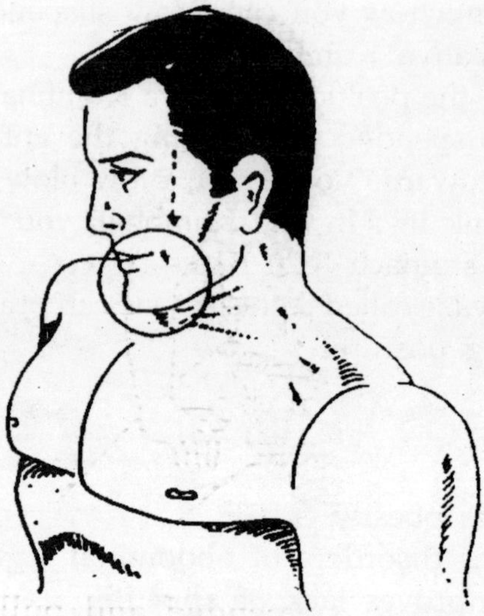

Stand erect with your feet one foot apart. Bend the knees a little and then slightly bend forward. Rest your palms with fingers spread on your thigh above the knees. Take a few deep breaths and then exhale forcefully. This is automatically practised. In these postures the chin is firmly pressed against the chest. This chin lock regulates the flow of blood to the heart, head, brain and neck. Jalandhar Bandh is also practised in combination with Mula Bandh.

## Uddiyana Bandh

It is a very powerful Bandh and a basic for regulating the flow of prana and awakening of Kundalini. Uddiyana involves the lifting of the diaphragm high up the chest and pulling up the abdominal organs towards the spine. It means to fly up . This Bandh makes the great bird of Prana fly towards the highest chakra Brahmarandhara or Sahasara. Inhale upto fill and exhale so as to empty your lungs completely.

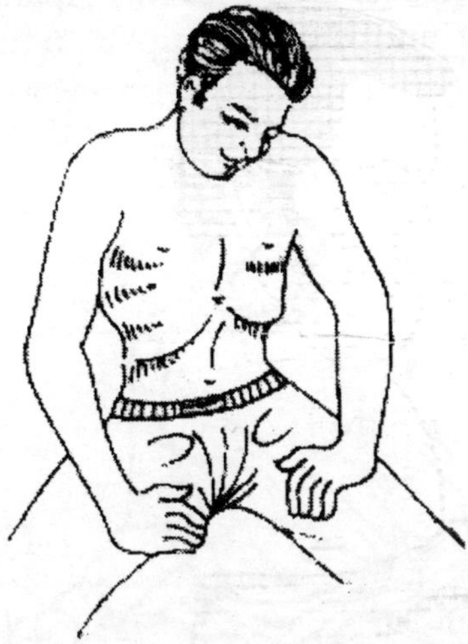

Keep the breath suspended and pull the entire abdominal region back towards your spine. Then draw it up toward thorax. Keep the pressure of your palms on the thighs all this time. Remain in the pose for 20-30 seconds according to your capacity.

Relax the grip on your abdominal region and inhale slowly and deeply. Repeat the cycle three to five times.

## Benefits

- Uddiyana Bandh is of great spiritual value as it forces the Prana upto Sushumna nadi.
- It invigorates the whole abdominal region.
- It is said to rejuvenate an old person, if it is properly and constantly practised.
- The uplifting of diaphragm massages the heart muscles.

## Mula Bandh

Mula literally means the root, source, foundation or the basis. In it the portion between anus and scrotum is contracted and raised. This prevents Apana escaping from the lower body and draws it up to unite with Prana.

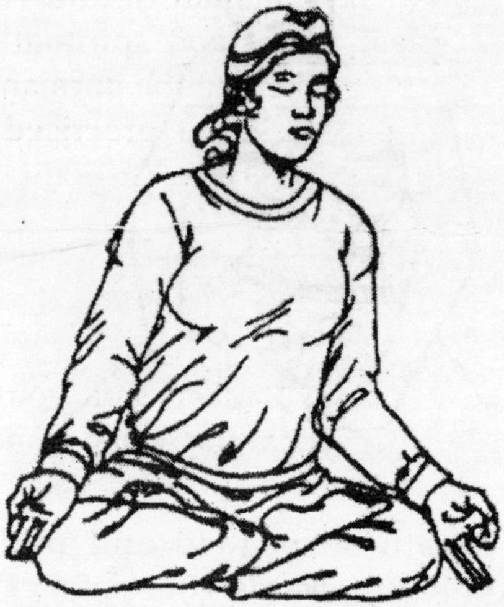

Sit in Padmasana or Sidhasan. Stretch your hands and fingers as if in Gyan mudra. Now inhale deeply and retain your breath. Press the chin against the chest in the chin lock. Now contract the region of lower abdomen between the anus and the navel towards you spine and pull it upwards towards the diaphragm. The contract and pull towards the abdominal muscles and remain in the posture for a few seconds. Now release the grip on abdominal muscles and remove the chin lock. Exhale slowly and evenly. Repeat the cycle three to five times.

## Benefits

- It cures piles.
- It cures the disorders of intestines
- It prevents Apana vayu (foul wind) escaping from the lower body and raw it to unite with the Prana vayu (the vital wind).

- it increases sexual retention power which we sublimated makes a man 'Urdhuvaretus' or a person of great moral and spiritual power.
- It also helps in awakening the dormant Kundalini.

The Mula Bandh should be practised when one becomes perfect in doing certain difficult asanas like Sirshansa. Sarvasana etc.

## Maha Bandh

Sit in Padmasana on a blanket. Shut your eyes. Now practise Jalandhar, Uddiyaana and Mula Bandh together.

## Benefits

- You get the benefit of all the three Bandhs at once by Maha Bandh.
- It cures the mentstural problems of ladies.
- It cures ovarian problems of ladies.
- It helps in strength mixing sex organs of males.

19

# Dietary And Juice Cure Of Osteoarthritis, Rheumatoid Artheritis, Backache

Juicing is itself nutritious. But for these problems, I have tried to elaborate proper diet and juices, which can be helpful for all sufferers.

## Osteoarthritis

Osteoarthritis is a form of arthritis affecting the bones and joints. It is characterized by mild early morning stiffness, stiffness after periods of rest, pain that is worse when the joint is used and loss of joint function. Symptoms can range from local tenderness, swelling of soft tissues, bony swelling and restricted mobility to cracking of joints in movement. Osteoarthritis is divided into two categories-primary and secondary. Primary osteoarthritis is a degenerative condition brought about by wear and tear on the body. Secondary osteoarthritis is brought about by predisposing factors such as trauma or previous inflammatory disease of the joint.

## General Recommendations

Osteoarthritis sufferers should achieve and maintain normal body weight. Excess weight places an added strain on the weight-bearing joints. For some individuals, symptoms disappear completely after weight loss.

## Dietary Modifications

- Try eliminating the nightshade family-tomatoes, peppers, potatoes, eggplant and tobacco. If symptoms improve even slightly, continue to avoid these foods. Though not proven, there is a theory that a long-term low-level consumption of the solanum. alkaloids found in this family inhibits normal collagen repair in the joints or encourages inflammatory degeneration of the joints,
- Avoid the citrus family-lemons, limes, oranges and grapefruits. This family, like the nightshade family, is thought to contribute to joint swelling.
- Avoid all refined foods such as white flour, white sugar and preserved and processed foods. Eat a nutritious diet that emphasizes whole grains, legumes (beans, split peas and lentils), seeds, nuts, vegetables, and fruits includes only a small portion of low-fat animal products.
- Significantly decrease your consumption of sweets and alcohol.
- Consider testing for food allergies.
- Check for hydrochloric acid deficiency. Seek medical advice in this regard.
- Try a juice fast, which has been shown to be very helpful for arthritis.

## Nutrients That Help

- Niacinamide may bring a noticeable improvement within two to six weeks. This nutrient is said to be especially beneficial for degenerative arthritis of the knee. (Waming! Niacinamide supplements may affect the liver or cause nausea.)
- Pantothenic acid may be helpful, as a deficiency of this nutrient has been associated with

osteoarthritis.

- Vitamin C may be beneficial.
- Vitamin E may produce effects similar to those of nonsteroidal anti-inflammatory drugs.
- Methionine is Important in cartilage structures.
- Superoxide dismutase may have therapeutic benefits.
- Copper may be helpful, as a deficiency of this nutrient has been associated with osteoa.
- Bioilavonolds have been shown to be beneficial.
- Bromelain has anti-inflammatory properties.

## Beneficial Juices

- Broccoli and kale-sources of pantothenic acid.
- Kale, parsley and spinach-sources of vitamin C.
- Spinach and carrot-sources of vitamin E.
- Carrot, ginger root and apple-sources of copper.
- Cherry and blueberry-sources of bioflavonoids.
- Pineapple--the only source of bromelain.

## Suggested Juicing Recipes for Osteoarthritis

### Digestive Special

Handful spinach
4-5 carrots, greens removed

Bunch up spinach and push carrots through hopper with

### Brocoli-Garlic Special

3 broccoli flowerets
1 garlic clove
4-5 carrots or 2 tomatoes
2 stalks celery
½ green pepper

Push broccoli and garlic through hopper with carrots or tomatoes. Follow with celery and green pepper.

### Blueberry-Grape Special

1 quart blueberries
1 medium bunch grapes
1/4-inch slice ginger root
Sparkling water

Push blueberries through hopper, followed by grapes and ginger. Pour juice into ice-filled glass. Fill glass to top with sparkling water.

### Pineapple-Ginger Special

1/4 pineapple. with skin

Push pirte apple through hopper.

### Ginger Hopper

1/4-inch slice ginger root
4-5 carrots, greens removed
1/2 apple, seeded

Push ginger through hopper with carrots and apple.

### Rheumatoid Arthritis

Rheumatoid arthritis is a systemic disease characterized by inflammatory changes in joints and related structures. Its symptoms include fatigue, low-grade fever, weakness joint stiffness and pain. There is often severe joint pain, with increased inflammation beginning In small Joints and progressively affecting all joints in the body. Evidence exists that rheumatoid arthritis is an auto immune reaction in which antibodies develop against components of joint tissues.

### Dietary Modifications

- Consume a low-fat, low-calorie diet excluding most animal sources (meat, dairy products and so forth). Studies have shown that patients following this type of diet experienced remission of joint symptoms. A vegetarian diet, excluding all animal sources but fish, has been found to be very beneficial.

- Increase your consumption of cold-water fish, e.g., mackerel. salmon tuna, and sardines. Cod-liver oil may also be beneficial.
- Exclude refined sugar, reflned wheat flour, cornflour, salt, strong spices. alcohol, tea and coffee from your diet.
- Identify food allergies.
- Check for low stomach acid (hydrochloric acid). See your doctor for testing.
- One folk remedy calls for drinking basil as a tea. Basil has been used to ease rheumatoid pain.
- Try a Juice fast, which has been shown to help arthritis.

## Nutrients That Help

- Vitamin C has anti-inflammatory action.
- Vitamin- E has anti-inflammatory action.
- Vitamin may stabilize the membranes and cells of rheumatoid tissue.
- Pantothenic acid may be helpful, as deficiencies of this nutrient have been found to be directly related to symptoms.
- Copper has anti-inflammatory action.
- Iron may be helpful, as an iron deficiency may be involved. (Supplementation is controversial. Food is the best source.)
- Manganese may have therapeutic benefits.
- Selenium may be helpful, as a deficiency may be involved.
- Sulphur may be helpful, as a deficiency may be invoived.

- Zinc may be helpful, as a deficiency may be involved.
- Bromelain has anti-inflammatory properties.
- Omega-3 fatty acids have therapeutic benefits.
- Superoxide dismutase has anti-inflammatory properties.

## Beneficial Juices

- Parsley, broccoli. and spinach-sources of vitamin C.
- Spinach, carrot, and tomato-sources of vitamin E.
- Broccoli, lettuce, and cabbage-sources of vitamin K.
- Broccoli and kale-sources of pantothenic acid.
- Carrot, ginger root and apple-sources of copper.
- Parsley, beet greens and broccoli-sources of iron.
- Spinach, beet greens, carrot, turnip, orange and grape-sources of manganese.
- Ginger root, parsley and carrot-sources of selenium.
- Cabbage and kale-sources of sulphur.
- Ginger root, parsley, garlic and carrot-sources of zinc.
- Pineapple-the only source of bromelain.
- Dark green vegetables-sources of omega-3 fatty acids.

## Suggested Juicing Recipes For Rheumatoid Arthritis

### Spinach-Carrot Special

Small handful spinach
4-5 carrots, greens removed
½ apple, seed

Bunch up spinach and push through hopper with carrots and apple.

## Garden Salad Special

3 broccoli flowerets
1 garlic clove
4-5 carrots or 2 tomatoes
2 stalks celery
Bromelain green pepper

Push broccoli and garlic through hopper with carrots or tornatoes. Follow with celery and green pepper

## Ginger-Carrot Special

1/4-inch slice ginger root
4-5 carrots, greens removed
¼ apple seeded

Push ginger through hopper with carrots and apple.

## Pineapple special

1/4 pineapple, with skin
½ apple, seeded
1/4-inch slice ginger root

Push pineapple through hopper with apple and ginger.

## Ginger Berry Special

1 quart blueberries
1 medium bunch grapes
Winch slice ginger root
Sparkling water

Push blueberries through hopper, followed by grapes and ginger. Pour juice into ice filed glass. FW glass to top with sparkling water.

## Potassium Broth

Handful parsley
Handful spinach
4-5 carrots, greens removed
2 stalks celery

Bunch up parsley and spinach leaves, and push through hopper with carrots and celery.

## Cleansing Cocktail

1/4-inch slice ginger root
1 beet
¼ apple, seeded
4 carrots. greens removed

Push ginger, beet and apple through hopper with carrots.

## Backache

Backache is a common syndrome characterized by pain and tenderness in the muscles or in the muscles' attachments to other regions, such as the sacroiliac. Back pain is a signal that something is wrong in the body. It can be caused by infection, disorders of the vertebral column, or a number of other conditions, -including stress. Back pain is a sign to take action and seek lorofessional medical advice. There are some things you can do in addition to help the healing process.

## General Recommendations

From a psychological standpoint, much can be done to help control back pain. For example, focusing, relaxation methods and biofeed back can all be very helpful. In addition, physical therapy, massage and acupuncture have provided therapeutic benefits. Diet may not have much influence on how one perceives back pain, but it can be very important in the healing process. An exception would be certain herbal remedies that have been used throughout history in the treatment of pain, such as red pepper, clove oil, German chamomile, and wintergreen oil. Traditionally, chestnuts also have been used to relieve backache.

## Dietary Modifications

- Reduce your consumption of animal fats. In

decreasing your consumption of these fats, you will decrease your intake of arachidonic acid, which contributes to the inflammatory process.

- Eat more fatty cold-waterfish, such as mackerel, herring, and salmon. These fish contain a substance that has anti-inflammatory properties.
- Avoid instant coffee. A study has shown that instant coffee blocks certain receptor sites in the brain that naturally help the body control pain. When these receptor sites are blocked, the body is more susceptible to pain.
- Follow one of the cleansing diets. Many people have experienced pain relief and healing from injuries during and after a cleansing diet. Cherie experienced a great deal of pain after a car accident In which she sustained whiplash injuries. After six months of therapy without much improvement, she went on a three-day juice fast, after which her condition greatly improved.

## Nutrients That Help

- Vitamin K has shown some promising results in pain management in studies not yet published.
- Copper deficiency can contribute to pain perception.
- D-phenylalaniwi, an amino acid, may effectively ease chronic pain even when medications offer no relief. Speak to your doctor about supplementation.

## Beneficial Juices

- Turnip greens, broccoli, lettuce, cabbage and spinach-sources of vitamin K.
- Carrot, garlic, and ginger root-sources of copper.

## Suggested Juicing Recipes For Backache

### Vegetables-Apple Special

| | |
|---|---|
| 2 lettuce leaves<br>1 small wedge cabbage<br>4-5 carrots, greens removed<br>3 broccoli flowerets<br>½ apple, seeded | Bunch up lettuce leaves and push through hopper with cabbage, carrots, broccoli, and apple. |

### Ginger Carrot Special

| | |
|---|---|
| ¼ inch slice ginger root<br>4-5 carrots, greens removed<br>½ apple, seeded | Push ginger through hopper with carrots and apple. |

### Ginger Apple Special

| | |
|---|---|
| 1/4-inch slice ginger root<br>1 apple, seeded<br>Sparkling water | Push ginger through hopper with apple. Pow-juice into ice-filled glass. Fill, glass to top with sparkling water. |

### Potassium Special

| | |
|---|---|
| Handful parsley<br>Handful spinach<br>4-5 carrots, greens removed<br>2 stalks celery | Bunch up parsley and spinach leaves, and push through hopper with carrots and celery. |

### Digestive Special

| | |
|---|---|
| Handful spinach<br>4-5 carrots, greens removed | Bunch up spinach and push through hopper with carrots. |

20

# Ayurvedic Treatment For Pains Of Muscles And Joints

In our daily life, we suffer from sprain, back ache and body aches. Here are the remedies for various muscular & joint disorders:-

## Muscular Cramps

- Apply clove oil on the affected parts.

## Sprain

- Chop raw onions and put in a towel. Place this over the sprain to relieve pain and bring down the swelling. Alternatively, make a footbath of lavender oil and water and soak your ankle, but do not massage the area.
- Grind lime leaves into a fine paste. Mix it with an equal quantity of butter. Apply on the affected areas.
- Mix equal parts of almonds oil & garlic oil and massage over the affected parts.
- Take 1 gram flour, just a pinchful, and add half of its quantity with equal amount of turmeric powder. Add linseed oil in it or any other oil like of mustard or til, and make the poultice . Apply it on the sprained portion. The poultice will enhance the blood circulation and in two days' time the relief will be there.

## Muscular Pain

- Warm the papaya leaf over the fire and apply on affected parts.
- Heat ginger (adrak) paste with turmeric (haldi) paste (1:1) and apply.
- Soak ½ teaspoon liquoric (mulathi) root powder in 1 cup water and leave overnight. Mix into the infusion 1 cup rice gruel (cooked broken rice) and take every morning.

## Rib Pain

- Grind a turmeric piece and mix in a hot water to form a thick paste. Apply this paste over the ribs aching. Soon the pain will vanish. In case you feel you are not having the desired effect, prepare the oil of turmeric and lightly massage your aching ribs with this oil. Another treatment for quick relief is to mix turmeric powder in the milk of the Aak plant (the medicinal plant, swallow wort, whose botanical name is Calotropes Gigantea) and apply over the ribs. This paste will quickly give relief.

## Ankle Swelling & Pain

- Mix equal quantities of castor oil and lime juice. Massage the affected area with the mixture. Also drink 1 cup warm water mixed with lime juice and honey.

## Heels Having Pain

- Mix equal amounts by weight of carom seeds (ajwain) onion seeds (kalaunji), fenugreek seeds (methi daana) and saboot isabgol. Have 1 tablespoon everyday first thing in the morning. If you can grind them slightly in the mixer - makes it more effective. This treatment takes a couple of months but is a sure shot remedy.

**Note:** Saboot isabgol, tiny very light pinkish particles, will be available with your grocer or if you request him he will get it for you from the wholesale market. Do not use the husk which is generally used by people for constipation as that is less effective but not harmful. If saboot isabgol is not available, husk can be used. It takes longer for the pain to go.

## Legs, Swelling And Pain

- Mix equal quantities of castor oil and lime juice. Massage the affected area with this mixture. Also drink 1 cup warm water mixed with lime juice and honey.

## Athletes's Foot

Keeping your feet clean and dry is enough to discourage the growth of this fungal infection. Remember, it is infectious and you must keep and wash your shoes, socks, and towel separately. To sooth the broken areas of your feet, simply soak them for 10 minutes in a foot-both of apple cider vinegar mixed with water.

## Foot Corns

- Tie a fresh slice of lemon over the corn (painful area) and keep it all night.
- Massage castor oil on the corns every morning and night before sleeping.
- Massage for 2-3 minutes so that the oil gets absorbed. In 3-4 weeks the corns will disappear.

- Mash 1-2 cloves (laung) & garlic (lahasun) and tie over the corns. Keep overnight.

## Sciatica

- Take just 10 gms. of turmeric and grind it in 100 gms. of cow's urine. Add about 25 gms. of castor oil to it and make the patient drink the whole lot. The patient will get relief. Alternatively make the patient inhale deeply the vapours emerging out of the large vessel in which jaggery is being prepared from the sugar cane juice. But the patient must keep his body covered with a heavy blanket. The more he sweats, the quicker he will be cured.

## Paralysis

- Boil a few leaves of tulsi in a tumblerful of water. When cool, strain and put this water in a bottle. Massage this water on the affected limbs. Continue this treatment for at least two weeks. This treatment, coupled with regular intake of the tulsi leaves as an alternative treatment along with other remedies is helpful in giving good results.

## Fainting

- A hot poultice of carom seeds (ajwain) may be used as dry fomentation for hands and feet.

## Fatigue

- Take a glass of grapefruit and lemon juice in equal parts to dispel fatigue and general tiredness after a days' work.

## Body Weakness

- Soak 8 to 10 almonds and 1 teaspoon rice overnight. Remove the outer skin of almonds. Grind into a fine paste. Mix in some milk and pinch of turmeric powder (haldi) . Boil and drink along with sugar candy (mishri) or ordinary sugar to taste.
- Sprinkle the following on a platter of mango slices; 1 teaspoon honey, a pinch of saffron (kesar), cardamom (chhoti illaichi) and rose water (gulab jal). Take twice daily.

## Exhaustion Due to Overwork

- Boil ¼ teaspoon powdered cardamom (chhoti illaichi) seeds in thin tea water and drink.

## Gout-Swelling

- Take 250 gms. of turmeric powder, 50 gms; Kuchala powder, 50gms; pigeon dung, 100 gms; castor oil and 250gms. til oil. Mix both the oils, add turmeric, kuchala and pigeons dung and boil. When the solid contents turn black, coot and strain the oil mixture. Add to it a cup of kerosene oil. Repeatedly massage this oil on your joints. Always massage the adjoining areas before massaging the swollen part. Like if you have to massage your knees, first massage the upper thigh and thigh joint before massaging the knees. This way the raw phlegm will be dissolved and not shifted to other portion. Try not to have constipation when you take this massage course.

## Gouty Pains

- Mix mustard oil and rectified alcohol (1 part oil to 40 parts alcohol) and use as a lotion.
- Make a poultice of ground fenugreek seeds (methi dana) use on the affected part.
- Equal quantities of Asparagus seeds (halong). Black cumin, fenugreek (methi) and Ajwain should be taken and swallowed every morning in dose of 3 grams. The remedies are also recommended for rheumatism and lumbago.

## Rheumatism

- Heat the leaves of the plant swallow wort (Aak in Hindi) and tie them over the affected joints.
- Grind the guava leaves to a paste form and apply on the affected joint.
- Take about 750 gms. of the root of Arand plant and boil it in 6kgs. of water. When it is reduced to 1/4th of its normal quantity, then add castor oil to it and boil again till whole of the water in the mixture evaporates leaving only the oily substance. Strain this oil through a fine muslin cloth and keep it preserved, in a glass bottle. Massage your limbs with this oil at least 15mts. before you go to have your bath. In case you do it after your bath, then tie cotton wads after the massage over the affected joints.
- Take 'Binaules', cut, grind and sieve them and boil in water, when only thick paste remains. Dry it and then tie it over your affected joints.

## Rheumatic Pain

- Boil 3 tablespoon powdered nutmeg (jaiphal) in

1 cup sesame oil (til ka tel). Cool and apply on affected parts.

- 2 to 3 teaspoon pepper powder is fried in 2 teaspoons sesame oil (til ka tel) until charred. When it is warm, it is applied on the affected areas and massaged lightly.
- A 3 inch piece of dried ginger is grinded with a grape sized piece of asafoetida (hing) in milk. The paste is applied on the affected area. The area is exposed to the sun for imparting warmth and heat.
- The patient must avoid fried eatables and sour foods like curds and alcohol, moong dal, meat soup, garlic, onions, bitter gourd, papaya and green bananas are the foods which help in controlling gout and rheumatic pain.

## Joint Pain

- Take equal quantities of asparagus seeds (shatavari), black cumin seeds (shah jeera), fenugreek (methi daana) seeds and carom seeds (ajwain). Powder and take 1/2 teaspoon every morning.
- Combine 6 teaspoons each of ginger (adrak) and caraway seeds along with 3 teaspoons of black pepper corns (saboot kali mirch) and grind into a fine powder. Have ½ teaspoon with water twice daily.
- Soak 1-2 teaspoons fenugreek seeds (methi daana) in a cup of curd overnight. Eat in the morning on an empty stomach or soak 1-2 teaspoons fenugreek seeds (methi daana) in 1 cup water overnight. Drink the water first thing in the morning and also eat the methi seeds.
- Take out 1 tablespoon juice of fresh leaves of bathua and drink every day on an empty stomach for 2-

3 months. Do not add anything to the juice and do not eat anything before and after, for 2 hours.

- Make a tea from papaya seeds and have 6-7 cups a day, for at least 2 weeks.
- Have 1-2 garlic (lahasun) cloves or 1 garlic, which has only 1 clove in a pod, first thing in the morning.
- Mix 1 teaspoon of dry amla powder with 2 teaspoons of jaggery (gur) and have it twice daily for a month.

## Arthritis

Extract the juice of carrots and add to it the juice of Karnphool (Dandelion). Have just 5 gms. of carrot juice and add only half of the quantity the juice of dandelion. Drink this combination regularly for at least 15 days for speedier relief. It is also advisable to rub Mahanarayani oil on the joints.

## Bed Sores

- Apply honey on the length and breadth of a banana leave and lie on it for a few hours. Ensure its contact with the affected parts.

## Body Pain

- Boil 3 tablespoons powdered nutmeg (jaiphal) in 1 cup sesame oil (til ka tel), coot it and apply on affected parts.

21

# Pain In Joints
# Homoeopathic Remedies

**Ammon Carb** : tearing pain in joints, in ankle, and bones of feet, worse evening, cold, wet weather and heat of bed.

**Angustura** : tension and stiffness in joints and muscles, worse walking.

**Kali-Bich** : shifting pain in joints, worse morning and cold.

**Kali-Sil** : feeling of stiffness and creeping in joints and limbs with desire to lie down, worse cold bath and open air.

**Kalm** : pain in right shoulder and hip shooting downward with feeling of tingling, numbness and coldness worse motion and open air.

**Kreos** : pain in joints, often in hips and knees, worse open air and rest.

**Lac Can** : when pain changes sides of the body.

**Lac. ac** : pain in joints particularly in shoulders, wrists and knees with copious urine and feeling of weekness.

**Euon** : pain in joints, more in ankles, worse evening and cool air.

**Magnol** : shifting pain in joints with feeling of numbness, worse morning, rest and damp-cold.

**Paraffin** : shifting, knife-like, tearing, wrenching or electric-like shocks in joints, more in ankles and soles, obstinate constipation, pains sometimes in alternation with stomach or heart trouble.

**Pinus-s :** pain in joints, more in finger joints with stiffness and cramps in calves, itching about joints).

**Radium :** severe pain in joints and limbs worse night, better by hot bath, open air, walking, pressure.

**Form-r :** pain in joints more on hips with stiffness and feeling of contraction, worse by cold damp; better after midnight, rubbing.

**Phos-ac. :** pain in joints and bones, loss of vital fluids-**China** worse night, better by warmth.

**Aur-Met. :** tearing pain in joints with profound despondency and disgust of life, worse cold and night.

**Bar-c. :** pain in joints in old age, blood pressure, better in open air

**Apoc. :** pain in joints, soles, toes, cramps, and heat in soles, tingling in toes.

## Particular Group of Joints and Limbs Affected

**Piper :** pain in the thumb joint, right arm, paralytic weakness in hand, worse thinking of it-Ox.ac.

**Lil.t. :** pain in hip, ankle, right arm, legs better in open air.

**Sol-lye. :** pain in right shoulder, arm : elbow, wrist and lumber region with tingling : worse jar, open air, motion better warm room.

**Guaic :** pain in shoulders, arms and hands, worse motion, heat, cold, wet, better by pressure.

**Arg-m :** pain in knee and elbow with copious urine, better in open air.

**Elat :** pain in knees, toes, fingers and thumbs worse cold damp.

**Hippom. :** weakness in knees and small joints.

**Kali-c. :** pain in hips, nates and thighs, worse cold, at about 3 a.m.

**Note:** 1. Gout involves or changes to chest–Colch.

2. Gout involves eyes Nux v., Bell., Rhus-tox., Puls., Acon.

3. Gout involves heart–Aur-m., Cact., Kalm., Colch., Spig., Benz-ac, lith-c., Abrot., Led., Acon., Naja.

4. Gout involves stomach–Hydroc-ac., Nux-m., Nux-v., Puls., Ant. c.

5. Gout involves throat–Colch., Merc-s, Bell., Acon.

6. Gout involves Piles–Abrot.

# 22

# SINGLE JOINTS AFFECTED: HOMOEOPATHIC REMEDIES

Homeopathy is a complete science. If your single joints are affected, try these homeopathic medicines, as per instructions, written separately

## Shoulders

**Abrot.** : pain in shoulders, worse cold air, rest. **Mag-c.** : pain in right shoulders, unable to raise arm-Phyt., Sang. c., Rhus-tox., Ferr. met worse rest and cold.

**Hyper** : pain in shoulders extending downward with tingling, creeping and numbness, worse cold damp.

**Inula** : pain in right shoulder and wrist with bronchitis and bearing down in female organs.

**Phyt.** : pain in right shoulder, worse night, motion and damp cold.

**Spirenth.** : pain in shoulders with swelling of veinsof hands.

**Stict-p.** : pain in right shoulder, with red swelling, worse change of temperature.

**Stront-c.** : pain in right shoulder, worse cold, when begins to move-change of temperature.

**Ferr-met.** : pain in left shoulder, worse at rest better by walking slowly.

**Coloc.** : pain in L shoulder, better by external pressure.

**Rhus-tox.** : pain in shoulders with sleeplessness, worse

at rest, damp cold, better during walking.

**Asper.** : pain in left shoulder, radiating downward with cardiac weakness.

**Onos.** : pain in left shoulder with feeling of weakness, worse jar, motion.

**Agar.** : pain in left shoulder and arm, worse damp cold, better slow walking.

**Sul.** : pain in left shoulder with heat in palms and soles, worse night, wet and wash.

**Pall** : pain in right shoulder and right hip often with ovarian trouble.

**Kalm.** : pain of erratic character with numbness and radiating downward, worse motion, on raising the arm.

## Knees

**Apis** : oedematous swelling with sore skin and stinging pain, worse touch, heat, better uncovering, open air, bath.

**Kali-c.** : swelling with stitching pain worse cold and at about 3 A.M; backache.

**Kali-iod.** : pain in knees with effusion, worse night and cold wet.

**Calc-c.** : swelling of knees in fatty constitution, with sweats on head and hands, worse cold damp.

**Calc-fl.** : pain and swelling of knees with rigidity, worse change of weather, rest, better heat and walking.

**Sal. ac.** : pain and swelling, sweats, worse touch, motion.

**Benz-ac** : pain and swelling, offensive urine worse on uncovering and open air.

**Rhodo.** : pain and swelling in right knee worse night, morning, cold wet, stormy weather).

**Mang. acet.** : swell, painful and itch, worse motion and cold wet.

**Rhus-tox** : pain with or without swelling, lumbago,

worse at rest, cold damp, better during walking.

**Cocc. I.** : pain and swelling worse when flexed.

**Arg. m.** : pain in knee, elbow with copious urine, better in open air.

**Melil.** : pain and numbness worse motion, damp cold, change of weather.

**Nat-c.** : pain and weakness in knees and ankles, with swelling of hands in the morning.

**Coloc.** : pain in left knee, better by pressure.

**Elat.** : pain in knees, toes, thumbs and fingers, worse cold damp.

**Hippom.** : paralytic weakness.

**Phyt.** : pain shooting, shifting, jerking, electric-like shocks, worse cold damp, night, motion.

**Caust.** : pain with contraction of tendons-Rhodo. better warmth and wet weather.

**Jac.** : pain in right knee with stiff muscles in the morning.

**Nat-c.** : hollow of the knee painful-Caust., Lith-c.

**Puls** : pain and swelling worse evening, warm room, on letting the affected limb hand down-Vip.

**Hips and Loins**

**Aesc.** : pain in hips and sacrum worse walking and stooping.

**Kali-iod.** : pain in hips at night.

**Staph.** : pain less in hip-joints, more in back and loins, worse morning before rising.

**Nat-s.** : pain in hip joints often in left side, worse stooping and damp cold.

**Guac.** : pain in hip jointss with heavy legs, worse motion.

**Hipp. ac.** : pain in hips, back and things worse right side.

**Starm.** : severe pain in left hip better warmth.

**Puls.** : pain in hip joints and loins worse evening, better motion.

**Caust.** : pain in left hip worse cold, walking better warmth.

**Kali-c.** : pain in right hip to knee, feels as if back and legs should give out, worse cold, at about 3 A.M. better walking.

**Card-m.** : pain in hip joints shooting down to buttocks and things.

**Iris.** : shifting pain in left hip, worse evening and at rest.

**Irid.** : pain in left hip to thigh with weak spine and kidney.

**Elat.** : pain in hips with diarrhoea.

**Ginseng.** : pain in loins with stiffness and heaviness in legs worse night.

**Chell.** : r. sided pain in hips, thighs and heels, better by pressure.

**Paraffin.** : pain in loins and spine, shooting down to inguinal region.

**Ruta.** : pain in loins with weakness in hips and things making one difficult to rise from seat, worse lying down, damp cold.

**Rhus-tox** : pain in loins with restlessness at night, when begins to move, worse damp cold, better walking.

**Berb. - v.** : pain in loins with urinary complaints, worse motion and standing.

**Am-m.** : lumbago worse sitting.

**Colch.** : lumbago, better rest and pressure.

**Lactusa** : pain in left loin, worse motion.

**Aloes** : lumbago alternates with headache and aggaravation of piles.

**Cobalt** : pain in back and sacrum worse sitting, better walking and lying down.

**Dios.** : back-ache worse stooping.

**Gnaphal.** : lumbago with numb feeling, better lying on back.

**Ankles**

**Med.** ankles easily turn when waling, sycotic history,

time passes slowly, i.e. melancholy mood.

**Nat-m.** ankles easily turn when walking, liability to take cold, craving for salt, easily tired, worse morning, better open air, cold bath.

**Calc-p.** ankles turn easily, effective calcium metabolism.

**Caust.** ankles easily turn when walking, with arthritic, rhematic and paralytic trouble.

**Cham.** ankles easily turn when walking during dentition period, easily excited to anger.

**Mang. acet.** ankles easily turn when walking, feels better on lying down painful swell and suppurate.

**Nat. ars.** the trouble is accompanied by nasal catarrh.

**Phos.** when patient is hot blooded, desires cool places and cool drinks.

**Ruta.** after sprains.

**Sil.** patient chilly with defective nutrition.

**Pinus.** weak ankles in rachitic children.

**Nat-C.** ankles easily sprained and dislocated.

**Nat-Chl.** weak ankles and knees, swelling of hands in the morning.

**Eucal.** pain and nodular swelling worse night.

**Euon.** pain in ankle worse evening better pressure.

**Guaco.** pain in ankle shooting upward-Visc, causing lameness, worse cold damp, movement better pressure.

**Prop.** pain in ankle with inability to stand;

**Stront-C.** ankle swollen, and painful, veins of hands enlarged, worse cold, on beginning to move.

**Verb.** neuralgic pain in left ankle.

**Led.** ankle swollen and painful better by cold application.

**Lith-c.** pain in ankle when moving about.

**Abrot.** swelling, emaciation on lower limbs, pricking pain, increased appetite, worse cold damp.

**Arg-m.** swelling of ankles in diabetic patients.

## Elbows

**Arg-m.** Oleum. j., Guaco, Visc. Wrists Hippem severe pain in wrist with feeling of weakness in hands and fingers.

**Plumb** : wrist so weak that unable to lift anything, better rubbing and pressure.

**Ruta** : pain, stiffness and gouty deposits in wrist, worse cold wet, rest.

**Bov** : weak wrist with inability to hold anything in hand.

**Viol-od** : pain in wrist worse cool air.

**Act-sp** : wrist red and swollen worse on movement.

**Caul** : pain in wrist in females.

**Cobalt** : pain in wrist with sexual disturbances.

**Abrot** : pricking pain, swelling and emaciation, worse cold and damp, night.

## Fingers and nails

**Am-m** : pain, shooting, ulcerative, tearing in tips of fingers often in toes also, worse evening.

**Bism** : tearing pain in tips of fingers under nails, gastric derangement.

**Berb. V.** : neuralgic pain under finger nails, swelling of finger joints, urinary complaints.

**Sec-c** : fingers and feet turn bluish, pain in finger tips with tingling and numbess better cold and rubbing.

**Sars** : burning on sides of tingers and toes ; ulceration around ends of fingers, cutting pain under nails.

**Elat** : pain in joints of fingers, and thumbs worse by wet and cold.

**Calc. f** : gouty deposits in finger-joints.

**El. ac.** : joints inflamed, feeling of splinter under nails, nails which crumble, worse warmth.

**Ginseng** : burning in tips of fingers.

**Oleand** : swelling, stiffness and burning of fingers,

sometimes veins of hands swollen.

**Pinus :** gouty pain in fingers joints.

**Ant-c :** pain in finger joints, worse heat and wetting, nails brittle–Graph., Sil.

**Am-c :** fingers swell when arms hanging down.

**Bor :** throbbing pain in tip of thumb.

**All-c :** fingers about nails painful.

**Colch :** finger tips numb and tingling.

**Eug :** skin recedes from the nails forming pus.

**Nat s :** swelling around roots of nails.

**Cycl :** Cramp-like contraction of right thumb and index finger.

**Hep-s :** finger joints swollen, and nail of great toe painful on slightest pressure.

**Piper-m :** pain in thumb joint.

**Primula-ver :** drawing pain in thumb and toe.

**Apis-m :** hands and finger tips numb.

**Graph :** deformity and pain in nails.

**Sil :** ingrowing of toe-nails.

**Psor :** psutules about finger nails.

## Toes

**Am-c :** Big toe swollen and painful, worse by cold wet.

**Benz-ac :** pain or lump or swelling in great toe, offensive urine, better uncovering.

**Bor :** burning in great toe. balls of toes inflamed, hot urine.

**Colch :** swelling of great toe with sensitiveness to touch worse motion.

**Daph :** right toe swollen and painful, pain shoots upto the abdomen and heart, worse cold air.

**Elat :** gouty pain in great toes-Gnaphal, worse damp cold.

**Hyper :** pain in toes or fingers, shooting upward with tingling, numbness and burning, worse damp cold.

**Plb** : pain in right big toe at night, worse touch.

**Prim-v** : pain in big toe and thumb.

**Led** : ball of great toe swollen with throbbing worse by heat.

**Rhodo** : pain and gouty swelling in great toe joint, better warmth, motion.

**Thall** : toes numb.

## Neck

**Rhodo** : pain in right side, stiff, worse morning. night wet, weather.

**Phyt** : stiff, worse morning, motion, cold damp.

**Cimic** : stiff, contraction, feeling, in females, worse morning and cold.

**Bell** : after exposure to cold-after cold wet.

**Rhus tox** : wet-effects, worse at rest.

**Agust** : stiff, cervical vertebrae involved.

**Cereus** : pain involving back, arms and fingers.

**How to take medicines** : Homoeopathic medicines for such problems should be started in low potencies like 6 or 30 - three to four drops three times a day for a week and if there is no response than you can take the selected medicines in 200 potency-four drops once in a week in early morning. If there is no responce than please consult an experienced and qualified homoeopathic doctor.

# 23

# HEADACHE–HOMOEOPATHIC TREATMENT

Homoeopathic medicines work on symptom similarity. You can find a suitable remedy according to your symptoms.

## Headache from Spine or Nape of Neck Goes Over Head

**Sang. Can. 200**–With flushes of heat and distended veins, of throbbing and lancinating nature, often begins in nape of neck or occiput and having come over head settles over eyes specially right side (Sit), wheezing in ears, nausea and vomiting ; < morning till evening, in the noon; > in open air, sleep, lying down, copious urination, vomiting, pressing head with hands, rest and quietness.

**Strontia C. 30**–With vertigo and flushes of heat on face of throbbing and pulsatmg nature, begins in nape of neck and spreads over head to eyes or upper jaw, increases and decreases gradually nausea, < morning, evening, cold, lying with low; > wrapping head warmly, in the sun.

**Silicea 200**-With sweaty head, of sharp, tearing nature, begins in spine and spreads over head settling over eyes specially right eye, scalp sore, and sensitive to touch, sometimes nausea and vomiting, < by physical and mental exertion, jarring, motion, open air; > covering the head warmly, copious urination.

**Phos. Ac. 200**-With weight on vertex caused by strain or study, grief or disappointed love ; often begins in nape of neck and spreads upward < least motion, morning, music, exertion; > lying down.

**Menyan. 200-**With pressure and weight on vertex, sometimes begins in nape of neck and spreads over head; hands and feet cold. < on ascending stairs, one side, after eating. jarring; > by hard pressure by hands, stooping, sitting.

**Iris. V. 30-**With throbhing and shooting, of bilious and periodical nature, begins in nape of neck and having spread over head settles in forehead, extending to right temple and dental nerves; often preceded by blurred vision which continues during pain, < cold air, coughIng, motion, rest, lying down, night, right side; > open air, continued slow motion.

**Spigelia 30-**With protruding and squeezed feeling in left eye, sometimes begins in back of head and settles over left eye, increases and decreases with the sun, < in day only, jarring, stooping, straining at stool, morning till noon, night; > cold, rest, pressure.

**Gelsemium 200-**With feeling of a band around head and heavy eyelids with desire to keep them closed, begins in cervical spine or occiput and sometime& extending to temples, ears, wing of nose and even chin, of throbbing, hammering nature, thick speech and preceded by blurred vision and followed by frequent and copius urination, < tobacco smoking, heat of sun; > lying down, rest, sleep, pressure, urination head on raised pillow.

**Cocc I. 200-**With vertigo and bandage feelings, begins in occiput and spreads to nape of neck or spine, thought or smell of food us numb and empty feeling, shutting and opening sensation, eyes protruding specially in left side, < eating, jars> drinking, lying on back of head, cold and open air, sitting, after sleep, coffee, tobacco> in carriage; > indoors, rest, warmth, quietness.

**Lac. C. 30 -** From occiput to forehead, changes sides, nausea-vomiting, relaxation alternating with contraction.

**Sec. C. 200** -Rising from back of head, dark bleeding from nose, pale face> by cold.

## Headache from Forehead Goes Upward

**Lac. D. 200-** With blurred vision and obstinate constipation of throbbing nature, begins in forehead and spreads upward to occiput nausea, vomiting, copious urine, < light, motion, morning, during menses; > pressure and bandaging head tightly.

**Oreod. 30-**Begins in orbit and spreads through brain to the base of occiput sometims to scapula or the spine or the ears, < 1. side, light; > closing eyes, silence and rest; constant aching in cervico-occipital region.

**Pic. Ac. 30** - Begins in forehead and spreads over head to occiput, extending to neck or spine, < stooping, motion and mental exertion; > pressure bandaging tightly, open air.

**Phytolacca 200** - With syphilitic taint, spreads upward, < in damp weather, > rest.

**Naja. 200-**With anxiety at heart (Calc. Ars., Cact), in left temple and teft orbital region, spreading upward to occiput, vomiting, < walking in the open air.

**Nat. Mur. 200-**With tendency to take cold and compressed feeling, sometimes begins in root of nose spreading upward to forehead, of throbbing, bursting, stitching and hammering nature; sometimes increases and decreases with the sun, eyes feel protruding nausea, vomiting; < on wilking in the morning, mental exertion (reading, writing, etc.), cold air, coughing and sneezing, looking fixedly; > sitting, lying quietly with raised head, sleep, perspiration, open air.

**Bufo. 200** - With flushes of heat, weight and pressure on vertex, wave of heat rising from solar plexus to the top of head in hysteric or epileptic patients, < light, > nose-bleed.

**Ruta G. 6** - Of pulsating and pressing nature,

sometimes begins in temporal regions and spreads to occiput, sometimes nail-driven feeling in head; < slightest eye-strain - reading, sewing, writing.

**Tuber. 200 -** In schoolgirls or tubercular patients or chronic headache on the verge of maniacal state, sometimes begins in r. eye and spreads to occiput, bandage feeling. < mental exertion.

**Bryonia 30 -** With constipation, thirst for large quantities of cold water, great dryness; sometimes begins in forehead and spreads over head to occiput; < motion, moving of eye balls, stooping, eating, right side, in the morning, > rest, lying quietly, nose-bleed.

**Onos. 30 -** Occipito-frontal headache often on I. side, in temples, often on I. side and in morning on waking; blurred vision.

**Paris quad. 6 -**Feeling as if-

Scalp contracted, bone being scraped. Soreness on head with sensitiveness and numbness. Pulling a string from eyes to occiput. Feeling of wright. Feeling of enlargement of head.

## Headache Extends to Any Part of Body

**Pulsatilla 30 -** With dryness without thirst, with desire for open air, of erratic or shifting nature, enlargement of veins sometimes stitching extending to face and teeth; temporal pain with lachrymation from the same sided eye, < evening and warmth; > open air, pressure, bandaging head tightly.

**Ipecac 30 -** With persistent nausea, with bruised or sore feeling in skull-bones, extends to teeth and root of tongue, > temporarily by vomiting.

**Rhodium 200 -** With tearful disposition, extends to eyes, ears, nose,teeth and sometimes shoulders and arms. Pain sometimes extends to shoulders or arms.

**Stell 2x -** With sleeplessness and eye-protruding feeling extends to temples and back of head, shifting pains throughout the body, < morning and motion, r. or I. side.

**Ferr. Met. 30** -With flushes of heat in face, vertigo and anaemia, of hammering, pulsating and throbbing nature; extends to teeth,veins of head swollen, scalp sore and painful, aversion to eating and drinking, cold extremities, < 1. side, after menses, after mid-night, lying down, > walking slowly, open air, pressure with hands.

**Arg. Nit. 200**-With feeling of fullness, heaviness, and enlargement, vertigo and buzzing in ears attack often ends in unconsciousness and bilious vomiting; pain extends to the corresponding eye; pain increases and decreases rapidly ; < often L. side, mental labour or emotion, dancing, > open air. pressure, bandaging head tightly.

**Ptelea 30** - With red face and sore feeling on scalp, accompanied by hepatic disorders, sometimes extends to the root of nose and temples, < motion and night.

Note :-Drs. hold high opinion about Ptelea for frontal headache when other remedies fail.

**Menthol 200** - Pain descends, to eye- balls, particularly L. eye, < option.

**Chion 30** - Frontal with gastro hepatic disorders, extends to temples, root of nose and over eyes, sometimes nausea, vomiting, < stooping and motion., jar.

**Euon 30**-With constipation and albuminous urine, with increased acidity, pain extends to eye-brows turning to backside, < r. or L side. evening, > pressure.

**Chin. Sulph 200** - With vertigo and distension of veins about head and neck, of pressing, tearing, throbbing and pulsating nature, extends to temples, < L. side, noon, morning till noon.

Note :- To be considered in malarial attacks.

**Senecio Aur. Q.** - With feeling of fullness and sneezing, extends over 1. eye and through I. temple, < after-noon.

**Cimicifuga 30** - With uterine trouble of shooting lancinating and throbbing nature, extends to in-and-over eyes, sometimes to shoulders and spine; feels shutting and opening in scalp, feels as if top of head will fly away < evening, afternoon, indoors, during menses, > lying down, open air, bending the head forward.

**Sepia 30 -** With uterine troubles, sensation of weight on vertex, of pressing, boring and throbbing nature, extends to L. eye and L. temple; terrible forenoon to night; indoors, motion, stooping, jarring, evening, turning eyes; sitting, > Rest, external pressure, closing eyes, after sleep, in darkness.

**Zinc Valero 30 -** With uterine or ovarian trouble, hiccough and sleeplessness, of piercing and stabbing nature, extends to spine, often in hysterical females.

**Valer 200 -** With cold feeling, of sticking, jerking, drawing, pressing and stupefying nature extends to the orbits, < evening, during rest, open air, > motion, indoors, change of position.

**Menthol. -** Frontal headache radiating to eye-balls and over frontal sinus with feeling of numbness and coldness in nose, deafness. < L. side.

## Miscellaneous Headaches

**Bell. 200 -** With throbbing of carotids and flushed face during cold, coryza and fever of any kind, sometimes in r. side only, < noise, jar, light, cold, evening and bending head forward, > closing eyes, pressure, wrapping.

**Scutell-** Frontal headache r. sided with aching to eyeballs as if pressed outwards and, < rest and night.

**Oreod-**Cervico occipital headache, nausea vomiting, colic, > in perfect quiet condition.

**Glon. 30 -** With flushed face and eye ball protruding-feeling, of throbbing and pulsating nature sometimes it is felt throughout the body, sometimes increases and decreases with the sun, < heat, motion, jar, bending head backward; > open air, fanning, uncovering, pressure, bandaging head tightly.

**Cact. 30 -** With a feeling of bandage about head, sensation, of weight on vertex, of throbbing and pulsating nature, distended blood-vessels, returns at the same time < r. side> eating, > pressure.

**Kali C. 200-** With lumbago and dryness of hair, of stiching nature particularly in temples, yawning one sided, < cold, open air, stooping, after midnight, morning; < raising the head.

**Kali Bic. 30 -** With sore feeling on the scalp, feeling of fulness which extends to the root of nose and angle of eye, one sided, preceded by blurred vision, which is > when headache increases, < morning till noon, on waking in the morning.

**Cann. Ind. 200 -** With talkativeness and forgetfulness, of throbbing nature with shutting and opening feeling in brain shocks in brain with shaking of head, heavy load feeling on head sometimes feeling as if cold water dropping on head, time and space seem long.

**Melif 30 -** With flushed face, blood-shot eyes and feeling of fulness all over head, of bursting and throbbing nature, retching and vomiting, sexual irritation < 9 A. M. till noon, afternoon, > copious urination, nose-bleed, menstrual flow, open air.

**Nux Vom. 200 -** With gastric derangement and feeling of chilliness, of bursting or tearing nature, retching with aversion to food, sometimes feels as if nail were driven in, < morning cold, eating, > rest and warm room (should be taken at bed time).

**Paul S.-**Headachc after tea, coffee or liquor.

**Ignatia 200-**With tearful disposition as a result of grief, of tearing and sticking nature, feels as if a nail were driven in, < from eye-strain and mental exertion, strong odour, liquor, stooping > changing position, lying on back and painful side.

**Coffea - 200 -** With nenous exhaustion and sleeplessness, of tearing nature, feels as if a nail were driven in. < after sleep, eating, morning, open air, > sitting quietly, in room.

**Thuja 6** - Often with sycotic history, one sided, feels as if a nail were driven in, particularly in r. temple and root of nose, < morning, evening, motion, > open air, uncovering the head, perspiration, looking upward, bending head backward.

**Agar. M. 200**-With desire to cover head warmly, pulsating and twitching in facial muscles, feels as if a nail were driven in or as if icy needles were piercing into head sometimes the trouble extends to the root of nose, < cold air, standing.

**Anac. 30** - With sexual irritation and irritability of mind, feels, as if a plug or nail were driven in < from exertion and excitement, > by eating.

**Tarent. 200** - With formication and restlessness, feels as if needles were piercing into brain, < touch, strong light, > rubbing.

**Ran B. 200** - With sleepiness, exhaustion and sense of enlargement of head, of bursting and pressing nature, < from change of temperature either from cold to warm or from warm to cold.

**China 1x**-(10 to 15 drops at a time), with flushed face of patients worn out from loss of animal fluids, of bursting and throbbing nature, pulsation in carotids, < lying or sitting; > walking or standing.

**Psor. 200**-With increased appetite during attack and tendency to catch cold, of hammering, boring, pulsating and pressing nature, bandage feeling around head, < change of weather, cold winds, stooping, moving the eyes, fast walking, > eating, wrapping the head.

**Merc. I Rub** - With pain in bones of face, < night.

**Aloes 30** - With heaviness in eyes compelling one to close them in those suffering from uterine or haemarhoidal trouble, headache alternates with lumbago < after stool on every foot-step < from cold applications.

**Stict. P. 30-** With pressure and fullness in forehead and at the root of nose, heat and soreness in eye-balls feels sometimes fioating in the air < change of temperature, > discharges.

**Zinc Met. 200 -** With fidgetiness in legs and confused dullness in mind after suppressed discharges or eruptions, of pressing , tearing, stupefying and drawing nature, < in sides, > by discharges and open air.

**Plat. 30 -** With numb feeling here and there, creeping and cold sensation, changeable temperament - hot and cool, gay and grief alternately, pain increases and decreases gradually < evening in room, at rest,>rubbing and open air.

**Mag. Mur. 30 -** With roaring and numb feeling, sweating of head, constipation with accumulation of water in mouth, milk disagrees, of griping, squeezing and bursting nature; < morning, open air, wrapping head warmly, pressure with hands.

**Sulphur 200 -** With feeling of burning heat buzzing and roaring > heaviness and fullness, great heat in palms and soles, <of burning and pressing and pulsating nature, -< noon, evening, night, > open air, external pressure.

**Asclep. Syr. lx-** With obstinate constipation and copious urination, with increased specific gravity, feels as if a pointed instrument is pierced through one temple to the other, increased urine and perspiration follow headache.

**Scutel. Lat. 6 -** (5 drops a dose) - Frontal and at base of brain with dreams and frequent urination, aching in eye-balls, "feels as if eyes are protruding. < right side, noise, odour, light > night, sleep.

**All. Cepa 30 -** With appearance of menses, < evening, warm room, > open air, when menses flow.

**Viola Od. 30-** With vertigo and burning in forehead.

**Sol. N. Q -** 20 to 40 drops a hysterical and epileptic patients.

**Rhamnus 1x-**With soreness and sensitiveness all over head, of bursting nature, in head, face and neck. constipation, < evening, bending forward, with every step.

**Lach 200 -** With septic states, bead and sensitiveness of the scalp, left sided, < on awaking.

**Cycl. 200 -** With flickering before eyes in anaemic - Women, menstrual disorder, < morning on waking, open air indoors.

**Poly. Pin.**-With pain in back, leg, ankle, < 10 a. m. to 3 p. m.

**Lob.Inf. 30 -** With perspilation, prostration and nausea, vomiting, from temple to temple, < afternoon to midnight.

**Sabad. 6 -** With dizziness and coryza; of pressing nature; often right sided, < from thinking intently or looking fixedly at one object, exertion or concentration > pressure and lying.

**Carb. An. 30-** With feeling. as if head is going to tear into pieces, < night when lying down > sitting up and hold it tightly.

**Crocus. S. 30-** With black stringy menstrual flow, of throbbing, pulsating nature, < before, during and after flow.

**Lit. T. 30. -** With uterine and cardiac irritation, 'hot and wild feeling, > open air.

**Tabac. 200 -** With persistent nausea and violent vomiting, followed by sweats, < morning till noon and subsides by sun-set > open cold air.

**Theriod. 30 -** Pain deep in brain, < least sound and least motion of head.

**Ant. C. 200-** With milky white coated tongue, < from the heat of the sun.

**Hyper. 6 -** With feeling of soreness in eyes, feels as if lifted up high in the air, effects of fall.

**Usnea Barbat-** (5 to 10 drops a dose)-With throbbing in carotids, feels as if eyes will protrude and temples burst.

Note: It is a remedy for neuralgic, periodical, congestive and sun-stroke headaches when Bell. and Glon. fail.

**Gauiacum 30-** Of rheumatic character spreading to face and neck.

# SOME OTHER BODY PAINS

# 24

# Abdominal Pain And Its Treatment

Abdominal pain, one of the most frequently occurring symptoms, may originate from any organ in the abdomen, like the stomach, intestines, appendix, gall bladder, pancreas and kidneys. There are number of causes for this and therefore, any patient of abdominal pain of recent onset requires early and thorough evaluation for accurate diagnosis. However, the commonest source of abdominal pain in the region of stomach and intestines is the gastointestinal tract which consists of the stomach and intestines because it deals with outside material, i.e. the food and drink we take. A little overeating may cause distension and indigestion. A spicy meal may lead to an increase in acid secretion and sour eructations. In these conditions some digestives or antacids are taken for relief. Very often flatulence, diarrhoea, dysentery, or an infection may produce spasms of the walls of the intestines causing a gripping type of pain called colic. This is a distressing situation and suitable measures for immediate relief are necessary.

Various house hold remedies like massage, hot water fomentation, churan, ajwain, jaljeera, and sometimes even purgatives are tried, but their success is usually limited. Therefore, the patient takes one of the preparations mentioned as pain killer which provides immediate relief. What is so special about these preparations that they provide such dramatic relief? It you look at the salts of any tablet, you will find that all the preparations contain an antispasmodic (which prevents spasm of the smooth muscle of the intestine). In addition, all these agents contain either a pain reliever or a sedative and some even contain a purgative. Such remedial measures may be effective in mitigating the colicky or intermittent type of pain. However, if it is frequent or of a dull constant nature, the physician must be consulted. Under such circumstances the continued and prolonged use of these drugs instead of improving the condition, may produce serious adverse effects. Since an antispasmodic is the most common ingredient of all these preparations, we will elaborate a little on it.

## Antispasmodics

These are atropine or its synthetic substitute (anticholinergic drugs) and are used for relieving the spasm of the muscles of the intestine. The actions of almost all these drugs are more or less the same. There are only slight differences in their potency or duration of action. There may be some adverse effects caused and precautions to be observed with these drugs.

## Combinations

After antispasmodics, the next common ingredient in all these preparations is a pain reliever. Some contain a sedative or a tranquillizer as well. Pain relievers may not be of much help unless the spasm is reduced. Undiagnosed pain precludes the use of phenolphthalein, a purgative, even if it is associated with constipation. Phenolphthalein itself aggravates gripping pain being irritant in nature. All these combinations have no greater value than the use of antispasmodics alone apart from increasing the cost and side effects. Some important drugs are Meftolspas, Proxyvon, Colimex, Cyclopam, Buscopan etc. Use only after taking advice from your paediatrician.

25

# STOMACHACHE & GAS WITH TREATMENT PLAN

The distress or stomach ache after eating is actually classified in two ways:

1. Distress appearing immediately after eating (postprandial distress): symptoms arise half an hour after a meal, such as abdominal bloating, distension, fullness or pressure.
2. Intestinal distress: Here symptoms usually start half an hour after eating and continue for several hours depending upon person to person. They may involve the stomach , small or large intestines with additional symptoms (to that of postprandial distress) such as abdominal pain and cramps and/ or anal flatus.

Excess of gas in stomach and intestines is quite distressing and it is due to the disordered intestinal movements which delays the passages of gases through the bowel. Drugs might provide a symptomatic relief in the following ways:

1. The active ingredients may lower the surface tension of the stomach contents to facilitate the action of digestive juices, which will speed up the digestion and the passage of food contents from the stomach into the intestines.
2. The active ingredients may speed up stomach

emptying by changing the stomach's acidity or increasing the contractions of smooth muscles of the stomach or by some other mechanisms.

The commonly available preparations, usually in combination, may contain the following ingredients:

**Antiflatulents:** Dimethicone (dimethypolysiloxane) and simethicone (a combination of dimethylpolysiloxanes and silica gel) act as antifoaming agent by reducing surface tension. The small mucous covered bubbles of gas (which hold air back) come close to each other, coalesce, and a large bubble is formed which is easily expelled out.

**Carminative Oils:** Peppermint, cumin, 'azovan' oils, etc. relax the muscles between oesophagus and stomach, increase the gastric secretions and churning in the stomach accelerate the passage of food from stomach.

**Antacids:** Magnesium trisilicate, light magnesium oxide, sodium carbonate etc. reduce gastric acidity.

**Sodium Bicarbonate:** It is a household baking soda (mitha-soda) which releases carbon dioxide as it interacts with acid in the stomach. It is useful for relieving distress after meal. Elderly patients above 60 should not consume more than a teaspoonful daily and if one is already on sodium or salt restricted diet, physician approval is necessary. In any case, this should not be used for more than a fortnight, unless a physican directs so.

**Charcoal:** Activated charcoal and wood charcoal can relieve bloating and other intestinal distress symptoms on account of its absorbent properties. However, it may bind a number of drugs and inactivate them for the same (absorbent) reason. Not more than 10g per day in divided doses would be safe for adults. So, for children the dose should be half.

26

# Menstrual Colic

When we refer to dysmenorrhoea, we imply painful menstruation and pain may precede (which often it does) a scant flow but subsidises as soon as flow becomes normal. Pain generally resembles a labour-like pain, when some young girls have been seen to faint even, under the stress and severity of attack. In certain ladies, it is utilised as an-excuse (though rare) to take lie from domestic rut and routine. But, whenever a lady says she has menstrual pain, there is hardly any reason to suspect and, thus, deny her rest and treatment.

It 'is repeated that colic, during menstrual period, is quite natural though, degree, intensity and duration of pain often vary, depending on health status of a lady. During puberty, irregular menstruation, scanty and vicarious flow, it is quite common in, thus, should be taken as - a normal and natural consequence. But, if the pain is persistent, severe and unbearable and affects normal" daily work, then the same should he treated forth with.

In anaemia, ladies menstrual flow is quite irregular and scanty. In such cases, attention should be directed to improving general health. When health has improved, severity and duration will eliminate. In order to raise Hb count in the blood, one should try to depend on natural foods (as already detailed earlier), in stead of taking recourse to tonics. Aim should be to raise the level of resistance by supportive measures.

Abdominal colic and menstrual colic need to be deduced in the former, there is constant gurgling and rumbling, and there is a feeling as if wind has here stuck up. Relief is felt when wind gets discharged but, in the latter type its seat seems to be uterus, it is either inflammatory or nervous in character which often resembles a labour pain and surfaces only at interval but is never constant. Pain is felt primarily in hips, loins, lower abdomen or/and lower limbs. It often precedes menstrual flow but subsides as soon as normal flow is restored. In some cases, it may appear after the menstrual course has already started. Not only these but there are other causes that trigger colic of this variety but, then each case has its own history as to onset, progress and decline which factors need to be investigated.

## Causes of Menstrual Colic

- General ill-health, poor diet, anaemia.
- Exposure to cold or damp conditions.
- Retarted, interrupted or irregular menstrual flow.
- Errors and indiscretions in living mode.
- Imprudent use of drugs during menstrual flow.
- Some intractable disease.

## General Symptoms

- Uneasiness and sense of well-being lost.
- Headache with or without constipation.
- Pain in lower abdomen and lower limbs.
- Irregular flow with pain.
- Pain in' hips, back, pubic area and feeling of general soreness.
- Lethargy and disinclination, to perform even daily chores.
- Swelling of breasts and feet

## Treatment

Any spasmodic or as directed by gynaecologist.

27

# Angina-Heart Pain

It is a painful or uncomfortable feeling in your chest, back, arm, neck or jaw. It is a warning signal that your heart is not getting enough oxygen rich blood to do it's job. It must be remembered that, angina is not a heart attack. It is a symptom of heart disease, which can lead to a heart attack.

## When does it happen?

- Angina usually happens when you are doing something active like climbing stairs or when you are upset. If angina starts occurring more frequently, lasts longer & causes more discomfort than usually, it is a sign that your heart problem is getting worse.

## What causes angina?

- The blood vessels that supply blood & oxygen to your heart are clogged with fatty material called plaque. The lack of blood & oxygen supply to the heart causes angina. The chances of developing angina are very high, if you have heart disease in your family, unhealthy habits like smoking, eating high fat food.

### How to diagnose angina?

- To help identify the cause of your discomfort, your doctor takes a medical history & does physical examination. You may need to have certain tests done such as electrocardiogram etc. These tests can give your doctor a more detailed information about the health of your heart.

# 28

# PAIN REDUCES PLEASURE OF SEX

After my children were born, I have not enjoyed sex at all. I am protected against getting pregnant again so I feel that's not a problem. Also, I enjoyed sex a lot before children. Sometimes I think its all in my head, that if I could let myself enjoy it I wouldn't feel any pain; yet I know there's something wrong down then. My gynaecologist has not been able to figure anything out.

This kind of report typifies a woman who is eager for a sexual experience but is finding each encounter to be more and more negative because of the intense pain she experiences during each sexual act. Pain during intercourse is technically called dyspareunia. It has a number of different sources. Whatever the source, when pain is experienced sexual enjoyment will be greatly reduced if not eliminated altogether.

## Pain and the New Bride

For the new bride who is a virgin it is not surprising if there is a small amount of pain. Most women experience at least a little. This can be due to the opening in the hymen being tight and small. In the great majority of situations it is due to a combination of newne, excitement and anxiety which prevents the woman from relaxing. When the necessary physical changes do not take place (the opening up and laying flat of the majora lips, plus lubrication), then entry is going to be more difficult and pain more intense. Entry under these conditions increases the pain and reduces the possibility of pleasure. Once the woman feels pain, tension is likely to set in. This tension will inhibit arousal and block any kind of release. While many couples begin in this way they usually get past the sequence quite quickly. But the sequence can be avoided to begin with.

If you are an engaged couple or if you counsel engaged couples, attending to a few small details will reduce much of the anxiety and potential for pain. First six weeks to two months before the wedding date the woman should be examined by gynaecologist or qualified general practitioner. In this experience the doctor should be able to communicate to her whether her physical anatomy is normal and whether there are any particular barriers of which she should be aware. The couple and the physician should discuss birth control methods.

In the weeks before the marriage, every time the bride-to-be takes a bath she should use her fingers to stretch the hymen until she can insert three fingers into the vagina and pull it apart slightly. This stretching procedure will prepare the vagina for entry and will also help the woman become familiar with some of the sensations of having the vagina stretched. As the wedding comes closer this might be done several times a day.

The couple should be encouraged to take along a lubricant that is not sticky (not Vaseline). K-Y jelly or Lubrifax are recommended for genital use. For use over the whole body as well as genitally, a nonallergic lotion without lanolin such as Allercreme is good. The couple should plan to use the lubricant for all entry experiences, whether they think they need it or not. The lubricant protects the woman In case she dries up during the excitement It also provides a distraction from the focus on the entry. A small amount of lubricant should be applied to the head and ridge of the penis and to the opening of the vagina.

A final word of instruction to the new bride and groom

is to move slowly. No matter how many times they tell themselves to proceed slowly they will still most likely move ahead too quickly. If a couple can plan to move into their first experience with a great deal of gentleness, patience, ease, and relaxation, they are most likely to create a positive beginning to a life of loving.

## Stress Brings Pain

All of us show our tension in our own unique way. Some women, as they experience tension surrounding the sexual experience, will tend to tighten up their genital muscles involuntarily. In fact, they may not even be aware that the tensing is happening Since this is counterproductive to a fulfilling and releasing sexual experience, It Is not surprising that these women end up frustrated. But even more than the frustration as a result of the tension, they may experience palm For example, If the tightening occurs before entry it may cause pain upon entry. Sharp, spasmodic contractions after entry may also cause pain. The extreme form of this tension is called vaginismus.

Vaginimus is the involuntmy tightening of the muscles In the outer third of the vagina which prevents the insertion of the penis. This contraction can be so severe that it is impossible to. insert even your small finger. It can become a permanent state rather than just occurring as a result of the Initiation of sex play. Because it is impossible for the man to enter, vaginismus is easily identified. Should this be your situation, consult a gynaecologist immediately and specifically explain your situation. If he or she is not familiar with the usual treatment procedures ask for a referral either to another physician or to a sex therapist. This professional must be competent to guide you in the use of a series of dilators which are graduated in size and designed to eliminate these involuntary spasms. Be encouraged that this condition is extremely responsive to treatment in a relatively brief period of time. However, there should be some attempt also to understand the events leading to the vaginismus so that his pattern will not be repeated.

Another source of pain due to tension occurs with lack of release. When a woman does not experience an orgasm, she may sense some painful sensations in the lower abdominal area and the lower back. As she has become aroused the whole reproductive system, including the vaginal area and the uterus has become congested with blood in preparation for the organic release. The contractions of the orgasm are designed to release it's congestion so that the blood which has fined the cavities can be drained. When there is an orgasm this process provides a great deal of pleasure. When the woman does not experience release, the whole pelvic area remains engorged, which may cause chronic pain. This pain is usually not intense, but is a dull, throbbing ache similar to lower back pain. The difference is that it feels like it is further inside the body. Obviously the best remedy for this pain is for a woman to allow herself to experience orgasm. -In consulting a physician or therapist it is crucial to identify when the pain occurs and thus determine if it is the result of lack of orgasmic release.

## Physically Based Pain

Infections and irritations will obviously reduce pleasure. Whether the infection is in the external genitalia, causing pain during clitoral stimulation, or Is inside the vagina, causing pain during Intercourse, it will hinder freedom and enjoyment. Any kind of infection should immediately be dealt with by a physician. Sexual activity should be limited according to the instruction of the physician. Sometimes an infection provides the opportunity for the couple to focus on the rest of the body for those often bypassed, special pleasures. Just because there is an infection does not mean the couple should abstain from all sexual activity. If it is comfortable for both, the man can be stimulated to orgasm at the end of a total body experience without ever having contact with the woman's genitals.

Irritations are troublesome because there is no specific identifiable disease present. Yet an irritated vaginal opening or vaginal barrel can cause as much distress and pain during love-making as an infection. The best antidote to irritation is the generous use of a lubricant. Some women experience a thinning of the vaginal walls. Sometimes this happens with age, particularly around the time of menopause because of a reduction of estrogen. If the walls of your vagina are thinning, again consult a physician to determine the cause and then always use a lubricant to reduce friction. Even if the walls of the vagina are becoming thin, pleasurable activity need not cease.

Pain can also be the result of tears either in the opening of the vagina or small cuts (fissures) inside the vagina itself. Tears in the hymen usually cause pain on entry. Some women can identify pain at a very specific spot inside the vagina. Their report usually goes something like this: "It feels as if it is in the lower left-hand comer about an inch inside the vagina and it hurts exactly the same way every time. I feel I can even reach in and put my finger on it" When the pain is this specific, it is usually not the result of tension or the thinning of the vaginal walls but rather the result of a small tear inside the vagina. Because of continued sexual activity and the moist environment, healing is slow. When consulting a physician be sure to identify the exact location of the pain. Show the doctor so that he can carefully warn it and determine the nature of the problem. As a rule these tears can be treated with an ointment.

Some women report pain only during deep thrusting.

There are three main sources of this kind of pain. The most commonly reported discomfort is the result of a lipped or retroverted uterus. When the muscles that suspend the uterus are weakened, the uterus drops so that the cervix, the opening to the uterus falls into the upper end of the vagina. As deep thrusting occurs the penis strikes the cervix, causing sharp, stabbing pain. It may cause a woman to cry out. Relief can be found immediately by a slight shift in position. For many women a small pillow or folded towel under the lower back (if she is under the man) will shift the uterus enough so that deep thrusting can be enjoyed.

Other internal pathologies such as endometriosis or a misplaced IUD can also cause pain upon deep thrusting.

Finally, there may be pain as an outgrowth of trauma from childbirth. One such pain occurs in the sensitive scars from the episiotomy, the incision that is made between the vagina and the rectum to assist the birth process. There also may be tears in the ligaments that hold the uterus in place, in the vaginal wall or around the opening of the vagina. Tears are more likely to occur with a difficult birth. This was true for us after the breech (feet first) delivery of our first child. For those resuming sexual activity after the birth of a child we would issue the same encouragement given to the newly married couple: move carefully and slowly, haste will only hurt; be generous with the lubricant.

## Managing Pain

Whenever you experience pain, the first thing you should do is talk about it with your husband. Never grit your teeth and bear it. Define exactly where the pain is located and when in the love-making process it occurs. Even before you get to the physidan you may be able to avoid the situations that cause the pain if you guide the penis for entry and shift positions to make adjustments.

Except for pain from deep thrusting, lubrication will almost always reduce some of the intensity, even if it is from an infection. Then, discover what is pleasurable and focus on that for the time being. Avoiding entry for a few love-making sessions may be necessary. It is important not to continue the activity that triggers the pain. Whenever a negative sensation like pain is associated with a pleasurable activity like sexual play or intercourse, the pleasurable event will begin to take on the negative feelings. Even after the physical reason for the pain has healed, a woman may continue to tense up or avoid the sexual activity that was linked with the pain. Her pulling away and tightening up has become a conditioned response. Sometimes the pain will continue because of the tension. In dealing with this, use the same approach as you would for any emotional hesitancy or avoidance. Begin gradually, letting the woman take the lead until the tension concerning the pain has been reduced.

An increasing number of women, particularly young women, are reporting pain during intercourse. If you are among these, seek help after talking about it with your partner. Pain does not have to be tolerated. In fact, pain cannot be allowed to continue If you are going to enjoy sexual pleasure.

29

# HOW TO TREAT THE BLUES?

- ☆ When you're feeling just tired, a hot bath or shower and bed might be just what you need.
- ☆ Raid the fridge. Sometimes a bit of fruit or a sandwich might just be what you need to cheer you up.
- ☆ Phone a friend. Make it someone who is a good listerner.
- ☆ Do some exercise. Exercise does put you on a high- and it costs you nothing.
- ☆ Go for a checkup. You may have some mineral shortage or slight chemical imbalance causing you to feel like this.
- ☆ Buy yourself something nice- a new magazine, cheese, soap, coffee or a muffin at your favourite coffee shop.
- ☆ Untidy homes are depressing do a cleanup.
- ☆ Just go to the movies a feelgood one or a thriller will be the best.
- ☆ Go for shopping- buy some new clothes for yourself. Experiment on trying out new outfits for yourself.
- ☆ Have a funtrip- preferably visit a hillstation or try out some adventurous sport like river rafting or treakking. You may feel more relaxed and fresh.

30

# ACCUPRESSURE POINTS TO RELIEVE DIFFERENT PAINS

Accepressure is a science where a uniform pressure is made on a specified point by finger or thumb or gimmy (a device) to relieve different problems, especialy pains. Here in this chapter you will find points in our hands and feet for different pains like backache, too thache, cervicalpain, wristpain, pain of extremities etc. By regular practice and firm belief, you can be able to get relief, though other measures may also be considered with this theropy.

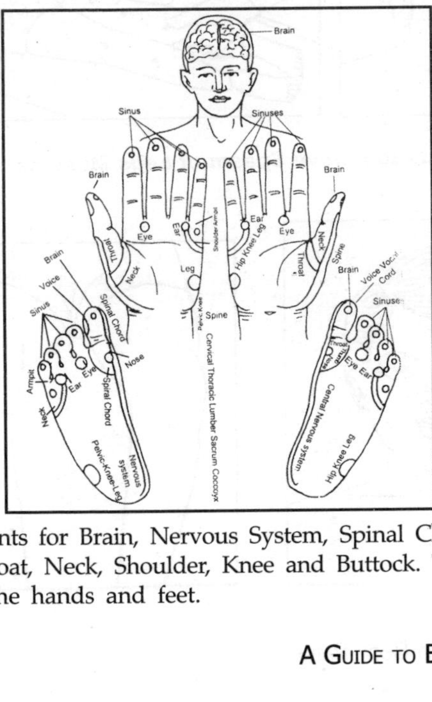


Reflex Points for Brain, Nervous System, Spinal Chord, Eye, Ear, Nose, Throat, Neck, Shoulder, Knee and Buttock. They are same on both the hands and feet.

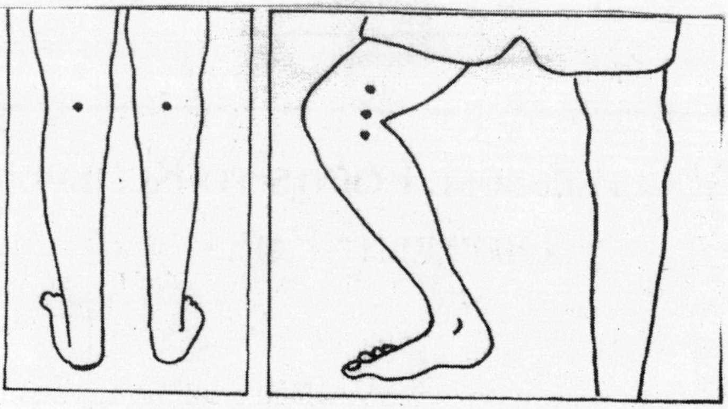

***Points to relieve Pain in Knees***

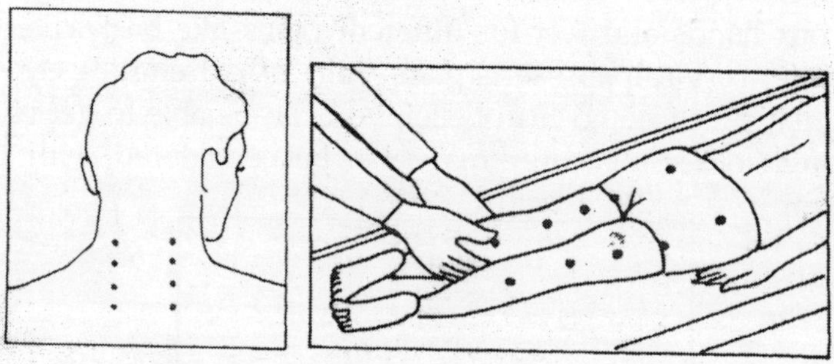

***Points to relieve Spasm of Legs Muscles***

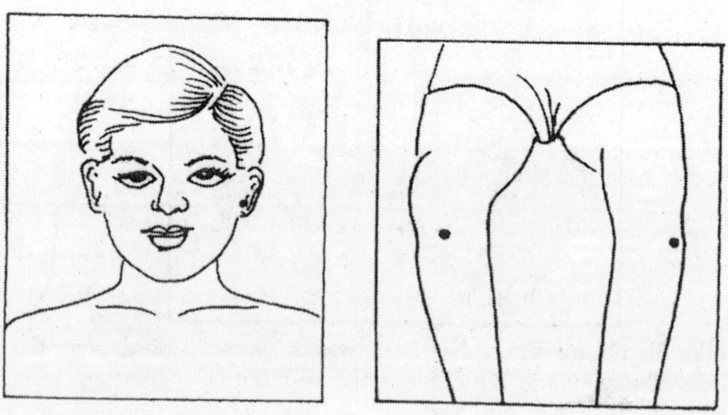

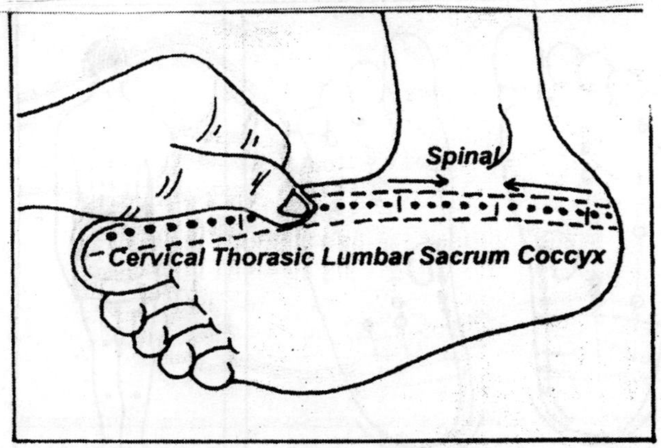


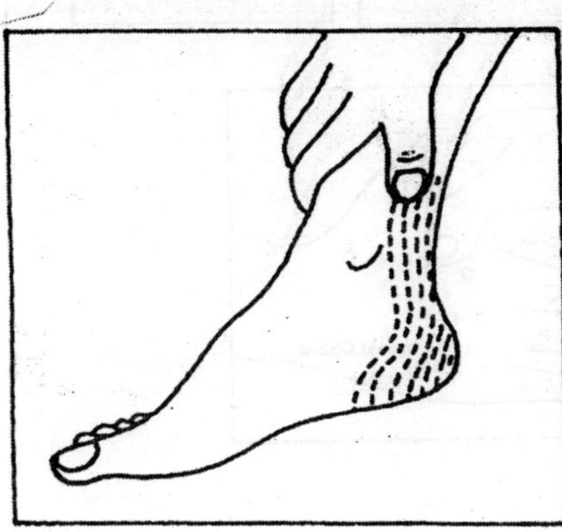

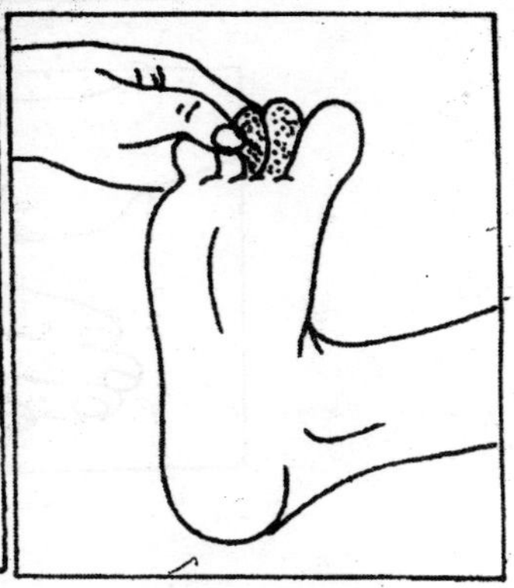

***Points to relieve Back, Hips Thighs, Legs and Heels***

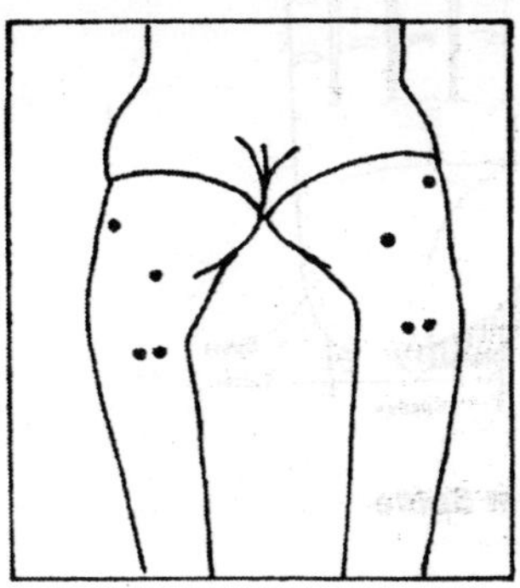

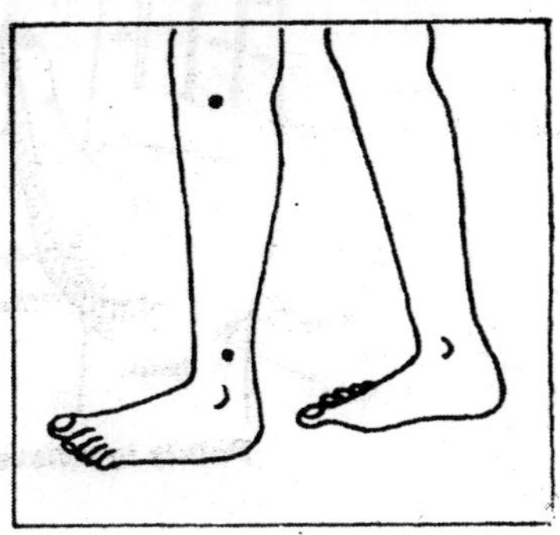

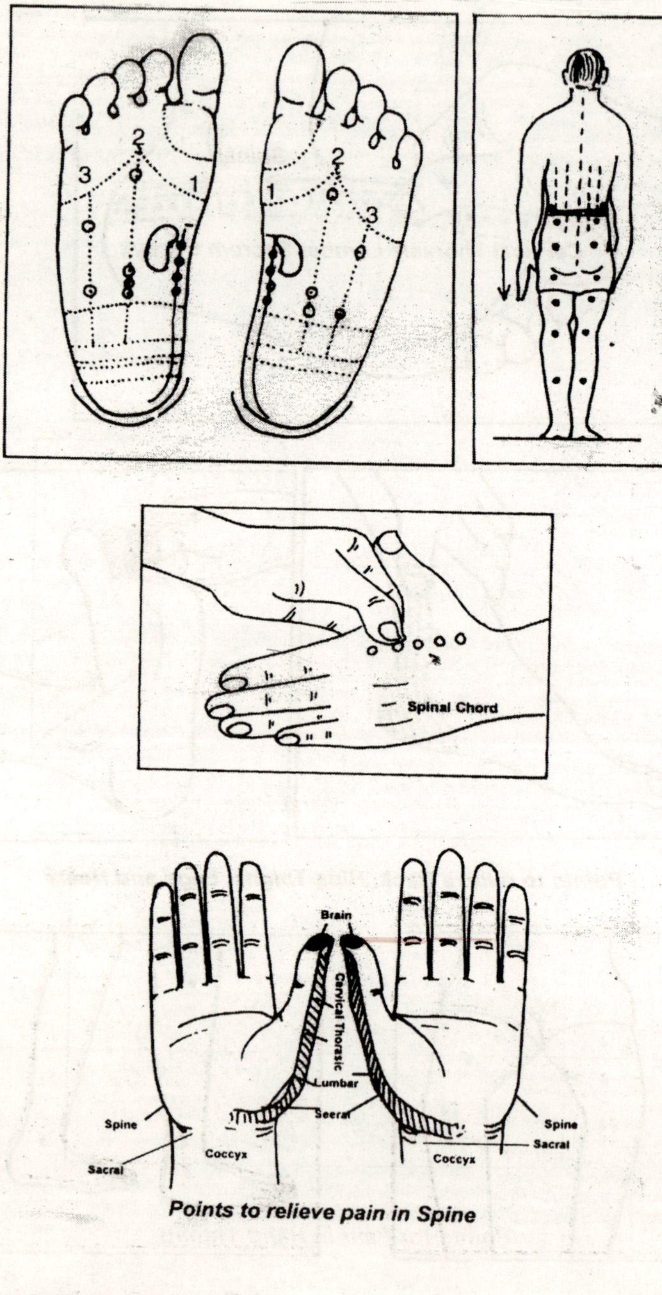


*Points to relieve pain in Spine*

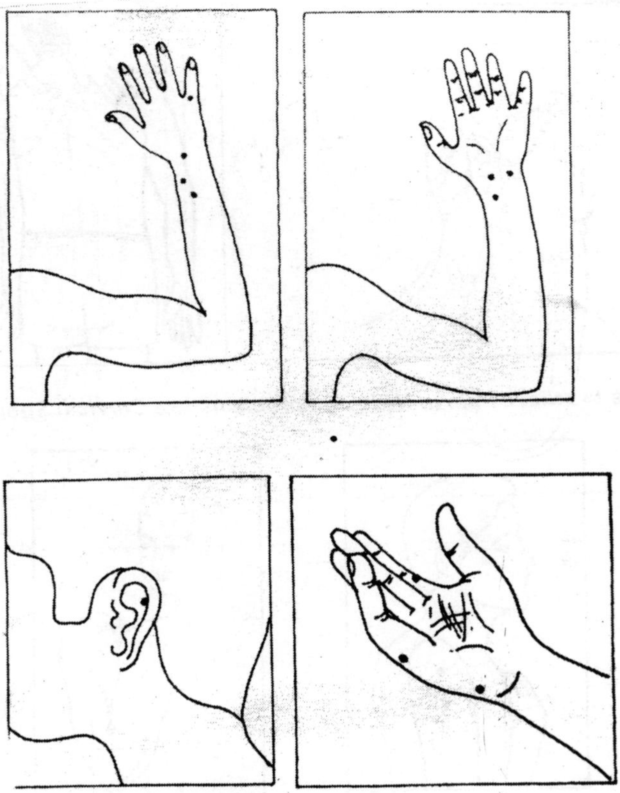

***Points for Wrist Pain***

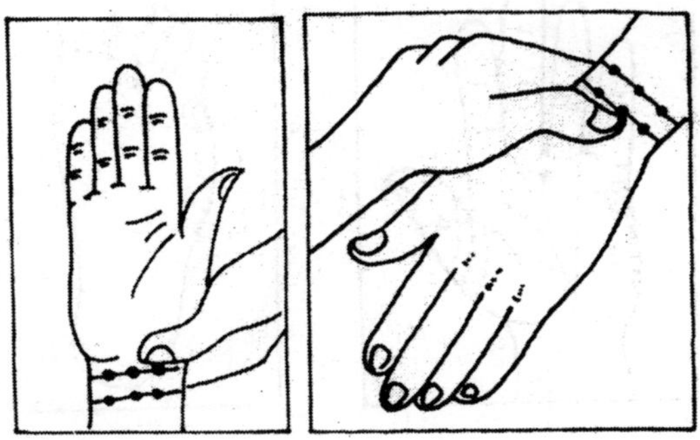

***Points for Pain in Hand Thumb***

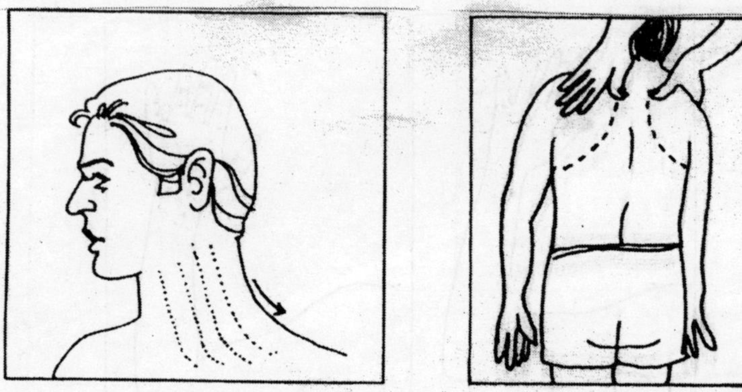

**Points to relieve Pain in Neck and problems like Cervical Spondylitis**

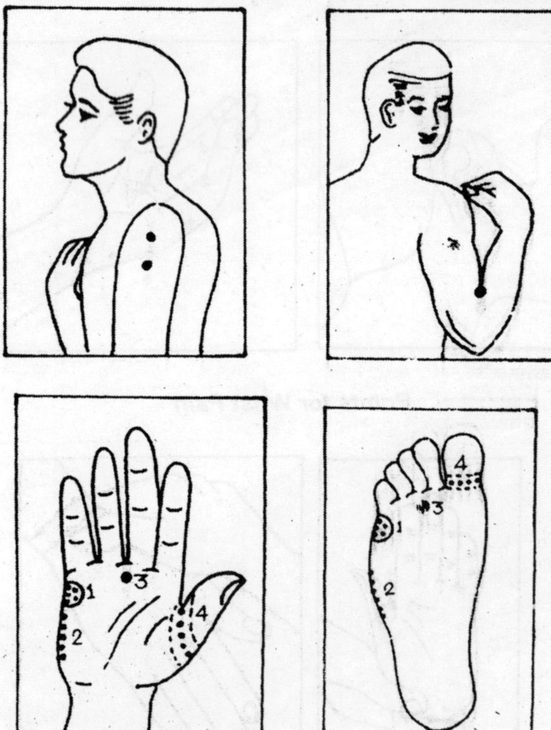


**Points for Shoulder Elbow Pain**

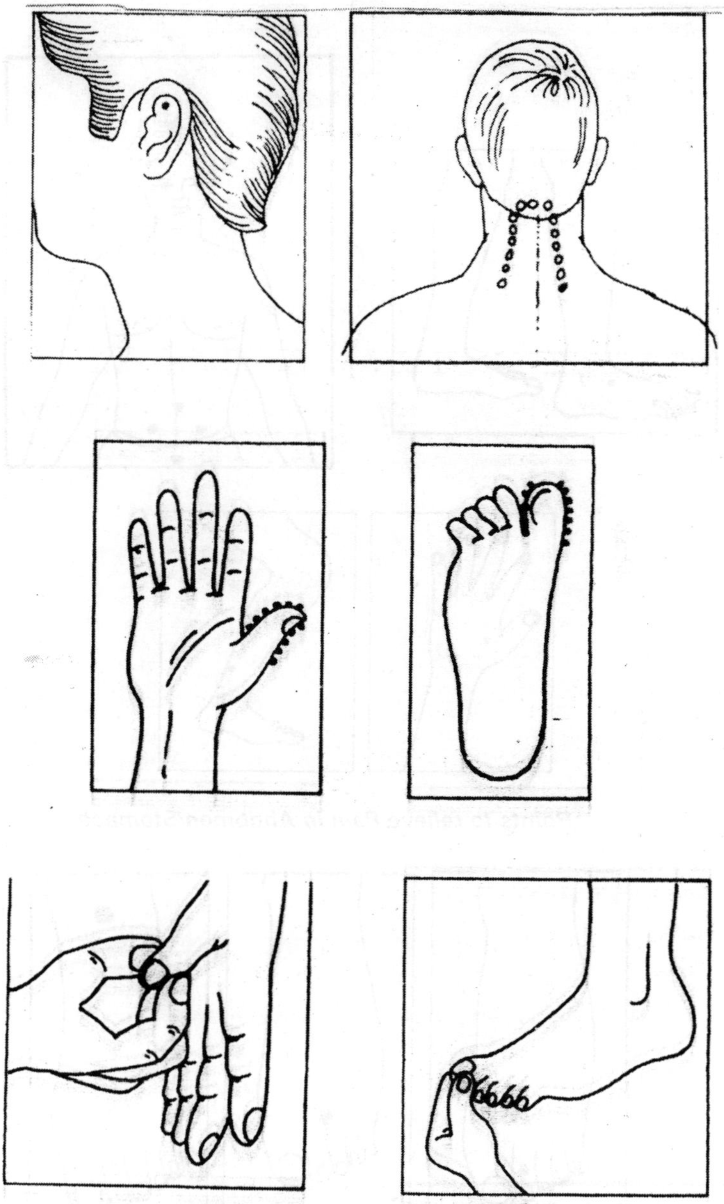

***Points to relieve pain in neck***

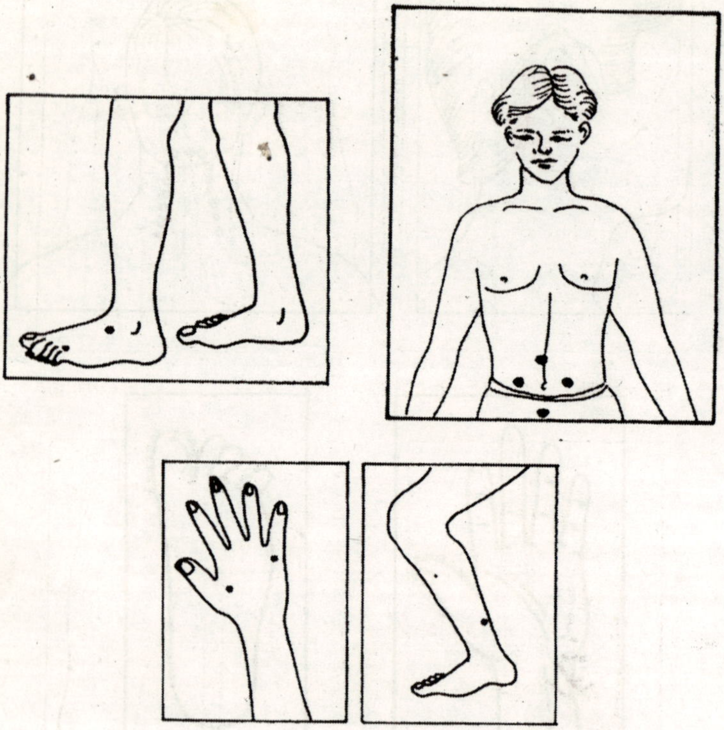

*Points to relieve Pain in Abdomen/Stomach*

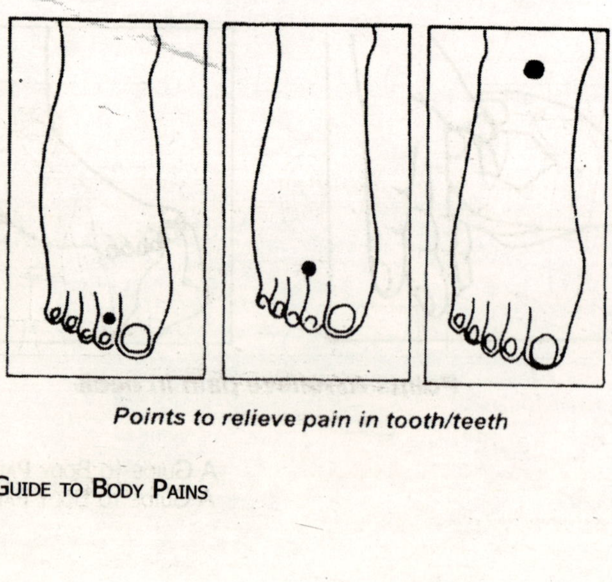

*Points to relieve pain in tooth/teeth*

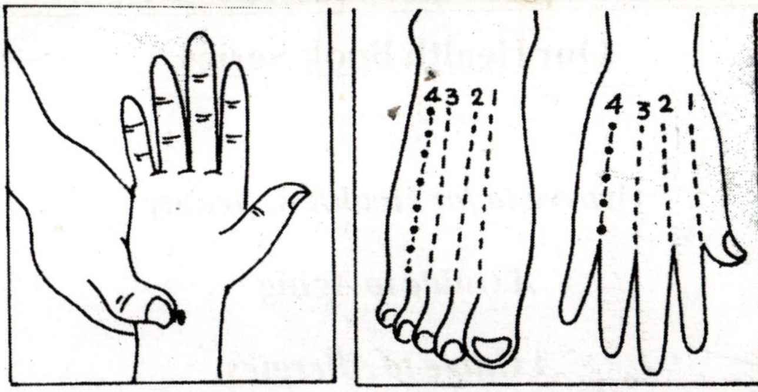


***Points to relieve Toothache/Pain in Jaw and Facial Neuralgia***

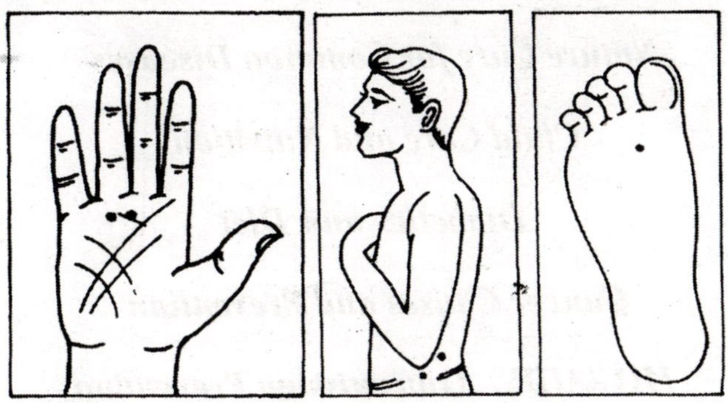

***Points to relieve Renal Pain***

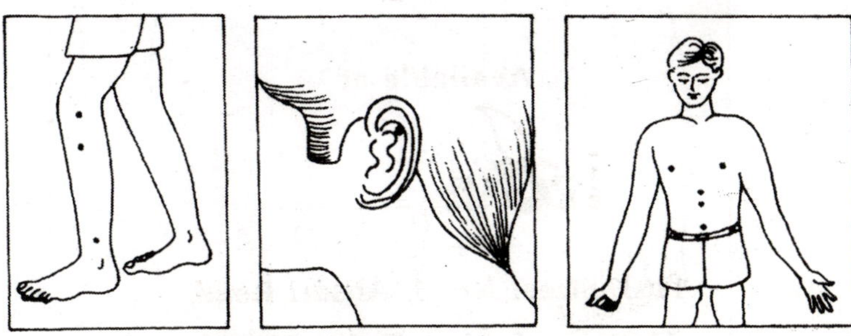

***Points to relieve Pain in Gall Bladder***